D1747763

Cancer and Aging. From Bench to Clinics

# Interdisciplinary Topics in Gerontology

Vol. 38

Series Editor

Tamas Fulop Sherbrooke, Que.

Cancer and Aging
From Bench to Clinics

Volume Editor

Martine Extermann Tampa, Fla.

8 figures, 2 in color, and 13 tables, 2013

KARGER

Basel · Freiburg · Paris · London · New York · New Delhi · Bangkok ·
Beijing · Tokyo · Kuala Lumpur · Singapore · Sydney

Martine Extermann, MD
Senior Adult Oncology Program
H. Lee Moffitt Cancer Center and Research Institute
University of South Florida
Tampa, Fla., USA

Library of Congress Cataloging-in-Publication Data

Cancer and aging: from bench to clinics / volume editor, Martine Extermann.
   p. ; cm. -- (Interdisciplinary topics in gerontology, ISSN 0074-1132; v. 38)
   Includes bibliographical references and indexes.
   ISBN 978-3-318-02306-0 (hard cover: alk. paper) -- ISBN 978-3-318-02307-7 (electronic version)
   I. Extermann, Martine. II. Series: Interdisciplinary topics in gerontology; v. 38. 0074-1132
   [DNLM: 1. Neoplasms. 2. Aged. 3. Aging. QZ 200]

616.99'4--dc23

2012043833

Bibliographic Indices. This publication is listed in bibliographic services, including Current Contents® and PubMed/MEDLINE.

Disclaimer. The statements, opinions and data contained in this publication are solely those of the individual authors and contributors and not of the publisher and the editor(s). The appearance of advertisements in the book is not a warranty, endorsement, or approval of the products or services advertised or of their effectiveness, quality or safety. The publisher and the editor(s) disclaim responsibility for any injury to persons or property resulting from any ideas, methods, instructions or products referred to in the content or advertisements.

Drug Dosage. The authors and the publisher have exerted every effort to ensure that drug selection and dosage set forth in this text are in accord with current recommendations and practice at the time of publication. However, in view of ongoing research, changes in government regulations, and the constant flow of information relating to drug therapy and drug reactions, the reader is urged to check the package insert for each drug for any change in indications and dosage and for added warnings and precautions. This is particularly important when the recommended agent is a new and/or infrequently employed drug.

All rights reserved. No part of this publication may be translated into other languages, reproduced or utilized in any form or by any means electronic or mechanical, including photocopying, recording, microcopying, or by any information storage and retrieval system, without permission in writing from the publisher.

© Copyright 2013 by S. Karger AG, P.O. Box, CH–4009 Basel (Switzerland)
www.karger.com
Printed in Switzerland on acid-free and non-aging paper (ISO 97069) by Reinhardt Druck, Basel
ISSN 0074–1132
e-ISSN 1662–3800
ISBN 978–3–318–02306–0
e-ISBN 978–3–318–02307–7

Contents

VII Preface
Extermann, M. (Tampa, Fla.)

1 Chronic Mechanistic Target of Rapamycin Inhibition: Preventing Cancer to Delay Aging, or Vice Versa?
Sharp, Z.D.; Curiel, T.J.; Livi, C.B. (San Antonio, Tex.)

17 Senescent Cells and Their Secretory Phenotype as Targets for Cancer Therapy
Velarde, M.C.; Demaria, M. (Novato, Calif.); Campisi, J. (Novato, Calif./Berkeley, Calif.)

28 Cancer Vaccination at Older Age
Gravekamp, C. (Bronx, N.Y.)

38 Immunology of Aging and Cancer Development
Fulop, T. (Sherbrooke); Larbi, A. (Singapore); Kotb, R. (Sherbrooke); Pawelec, G. (Tuebingen)

49 Metabolic Syndrome and Cancer: From Bedside to Bench and Back
Extermann, M. (Tampa, Fla.)

61 Frailty: A Common Pathway in Aging and Cancer
Balducci, L. (Tampa, Fla.)

73 Targeting Age-Related Changes in the Biology of Acute Myeloid Leukemia: Is the Patient Seeing the Progress?
Vey, N. (Marseille)

85 Comprehensive Geriatric Assessment in Oncology
Mohile, S.G.; Magnuson, A. (Rochester, N.Y.)

104 Pharmacology of Aging and Cancer: How Useful Are Pharmacokinetic Tests?
Lichtman, S.M. (Commack, N.Y./New York, N.Y.)

124 Surgery in Older Cancer Patients – Recent Results and New Techniques: Worth the Investment?
van Leeuwen, B.L.; Huisman, M.G. (Groningen); Audisio, R.A. (St. Helens)

132 Organizing the Geriatrician/Oncologist Partnership: One Size Fits All? Practical Solutions
Holmes, H.M. (Houston, Tex.); Albrand, G. (Francheville)

139 Geriatric Oncology Nursing: Beyond Standard Care
Overcash, J. (Columbus, Ohio)

146 Exercise for Older Cancer Patients: Feasible and Helpful?
Klepin, H.D. (Winston-Salem, N.C.); Mohile, S.G. (Rochester, N.Y.);
Mihalko, S. (Winston-Salem, N.C.)

158 Aging and Cancer – Addressing a Nation's Challenge
Bréchot, J.-M.; Le Quellec-Nathan, M.; Buzyn, A. (Boulogne-Billancourt)

165 Author Index
166 Subject Index

Preface

As I write this preface, I am just back from an exciting 12th Annual Conference of the International Society of Geriatric Oncology (SIOG). The conference spanned everything from basic science to public health and caregiving. These are great times for geriatric oncology as our field expands in all directions. This issue of the *Interdisciplinary Topics in Gerontology* series will, I hope, convey to you this excitement.

We start at the bench, with a chapter by Sharp et al., from San Antonio, Tex., USA, on mTOR inhibition. This is an important pathway in both aging and cancer, and the recent availability of mTOR inhibitors for clinical use in oncology opens a wide array of possibilities for interactive cancer and aging studies. We then explore how the tumor microenvironment can be altered by senescent cells with Velarde et al., from Berkeley, Calif., a group that has done a lot of work on the topic. We continue with two thorough chapters on immune senescence and how it affects cancer vaccine response (Gravekamp), and cancer development (Fulop et al.).

We then transition to a case example in translational research, namely the impact of the metabolic syndrome, which affects 40% of older Americans, on cancer development and prognosis. This illustrates an important development in our understanding of the interactions between comorbidity and cancer. Comorbidity used to be seen as mostly a competing cause of death, or something reducing tolerance to cancer treatment. Increasingly, however, we realize that comorbidities and their treatment can influence the behavior of the cancer itself, worsening or improving its prognosis. Dr. Balducci shares with us his expertise on frailty in the next chapter, another topic that links biology and clinic, and a hotly debated one in geriatrics. AML has a poor prognosis in the elderly, and numerous translational research studies target patients above the age of 60. Are we seeing progress? Dr. Vey tackles this question.

A key feature of geriatric oncology, like geriatrics in general, is its multidisciplinarity. A comprehensive geriatric assessment and intervention is at the core of geriatric medicine and Dr. Mohile reviews the state of the art in adapting this approach to the older cancer patient. Several pharmacokinetic tests are offered to improve chemotherapy dosing in cancer patients. How helpful are they in the elderly? Dr. Lichtman weighs in. Van Leuwen et al. appraise the role of the new surgery techniques in improving the care of older cancer patients. Bringing multidisciplinary teams together raises multiple practical organizational questions. Therefore our three next chapters explore how geriatricians and oncologists can interact (Holmes and Albrand), how geriatric oncology nursing differs from oncology nursing as usual (Overcash), and how exercise programs can be implemented for older cancer patients (Klepin et al.).

Ultimately, if geriatric oncology is to benefit the entire population, it has to be organized on a large scale. Bréchot et al. share with us how the French National Cancer Institute has been instrumental and deliberate in building up the geriatric oncology capacity in France. Inspirational lessons for all of us.

I hope you will enjoy the reading, and even more, find a multitude of ideas to feed your research and practice, and foster your excitement for geriatric oncology. Who knows, you might contribute your experience to the next SIOG meeting… Good reading!

Martine Extermann
Tampa, Fla., USA

Chronic Mechanistic Target of Rapamycin Inhibition: Preventing Cancer to Delay Aging, or Vice Versa?

Zelton Dave Sharp[a,c,d] · Tyler Jay Curiel[b–d] · Carolina Becker Livi[a,c,d]

[a]Department of Molecular Medicine, Institute of Biotechnology, [b]Department of Medicine/Hematology and Medical Oncology, [c]Barshop Institute for Longevity and Aging Studies, and [d]Cancer Therapy and Research Center, The University of Texas Health Science Center at San Antonio, San Antonio, Tex., USA

Abstract

Cancer and aging appear to be inexorably linked, yet approaches to ameliorate them in concert are lacking. Although not (easily) feasible in humans, years of preclinical research show that diet and growth factor restriction each successfully address cancer and aging together. Chronic treatment of genetically heterogeneous mice with an enteric formulation of rapamycin (eRapa) extended maximum lifespan of both genders when started in mid or late life. In part, cancer amelioration in treated mice suggested that long-term eRapa, like diet restriction, could be a pharmacological approach feasible for use in the clinic. We review the current understanding of the role of the mechanistic target of rapamycin (mTOR) in cancer and aging. We also discuss the tumor immune surveillance system, and the need for a better understanding of its responses to mTOR inhibitors. We also address the issue of the misperception that rapamycin is a potent immunosuppressant. Finally, we review the current state of mTOR inhibitors in the cancer clinic. Because of the burgeoning elderly population most at risk for cancer, there is a great need for our eRapa findings to be a proof of concept for the development of new and more comprehensive approaches to cancer prevention that are safe and also mitigate other deleterious effects of aging.

Copyright © 2013 S. Karger AG, Basel

If we could magically cure all cancers, would this in fact address the aging problem? While true to a certain extent, attacking cancer without addressing aging is an economically shortsighted and questionable health policy. If we eliminated all adult cancers, the overall cost of healthcare would rise by 7.4% [1]. The 3- to 4-year extension of average lifespan would result in more healthcare dollars being spent treating other age-related diseases (e.g., Alzheimer disease, atherosclerosis, and diseases associated with immune senescence, to mention a few). This increase in healthcare cost also applies to other age-related diseases such as heart disease, the elimination of which would increase lifespan on average by 5.2 years and health costs by 8% [1]. Ignorance of these paradoxical economic effects of extending lifespan contributes to the burgeoning cost of healthcare for the fastest growing segment of the US population (>65 years = 70 million individuals or a 20% increase by 2030; cf. http://www.aoa.gov/AoARoot/Aging_Statistics/future_growth/future_growth.aspx#age).

It is thus imperative that we address the following questions: (1) Can we develop strategies to prevent cancer while mitigating the diseases associated with increased lifespan, and (2) can we do both at the same time, with one or a combination of intervention(s)?

At the same time, however, we must also address two potential barriers to this approach. First, a culture that promotes a 'war on cancer,' centered almost entirely on treatment ignores the role of aging in the disease process. Second, there is a misconception that cancer is a disease while aging is not – that they should not be conflated. Contrary evidence suggests that, by far, age is the most significant risk factor for a wide range of diseases [2] (including cancer [3]), which consume enormous amounts of time, energy and resources. A tenet of aging research posits that age-delaying interventions also delay and/or reduce the incidence and severity of age-associated diseases. Cancer and aging, then, must be considered alongside one another to make meaningful progress in the mitigation of the disease.

Can these barriers be surmounted so that we can begin to meet the formidable challenge of preventing and treating cancer in a manner that takes into account issues of aging? We think the answer is 'yes', which on the surface appears fanciful. However, researchers in the aging field have, for a long time, been demonstrating that it is possible to delay aging and its associated diseases. We are referring to the huge body of preclinical work showing that reducing dietary (caloric) intake improves most measures of health, including delaying and/or preventing cancer [4], and, in the process contributes to the increase in maximum lifespan [5]. An increase in maximum lifespan occurs if cancer and other competing causes of mortality are all reduced (cf. D.E. Harrison: http://research.jax.org/faculty/harrison/ger1vLifespan1.html). Pituitary dwarf mice also exhibit an extension in maximum lifespan [reviewed in 6], and exhibit reduced cancer [7, 8]. Unfortunately however, translating these interventions to humans is not (easily) feasible in people. Is there a realistic way to mimic these conditions to achieve the same outcome in humans?

To get at this question it is useful to know what exactly the connection between aging and cancer is. Aging and age-related diseases (including cancer) probably share common underlying etiologic mechanisms. Currently, it is generally accepted that a continuing accumulation of damaged or aggregate macromolecules in somatic organs/tissues is an underlying mechanism driving the aging process, and is also presumed to be an overlapping factor in the cause of many of the age-associated diseases. It is argued that the elderly have more cancer (up to a point) because they have had a greater lifetime exposure to carcinogenic insults than the young. However, growing evidence indicates that aging in itself is an independent risk factor. For example, the development of cancer is about 50-fold more rapid in mice than humans, which closely parallels the difference in lifespan between these two species [9]. Campisi [10] proposes that aging senescent cells contribute to microenvironmental conditions that promote cancer. Importantly and discussed above, interventions that retard aging also retard cancer and decrease the incidence and/or severity of most types of cancer.

The proportion of elderly individuals in the population continues to explode in the 21st century making understanding the aging/cancer connection a pressing problem. By the year 2030, projections show that 20% of the population in the USA will be over the age of 65 [11]. Projections also indicate that the number of people over the age of 65 and 85 doubles in the USA to 72 and 10 million, respectively; after 2030 the oldest of the old will be the most rapidly expanding population [12].

In 2009, Jemal et al. [13] estimated the diagnosis of 1,479,350 new cancer cases associated with 562,340 deaths. Significantly, 60% of the cancer incidence and 70% of related mortality will occur in people 65 and over [13]. For the burgeoning over 65 generation, these data indicate that cancer-related problems will be significant. Because persons over 65 years of age have an age-adjusted cancer mortality rate 15 times greater than young people, the risk of developing cancer and dying from it becomes very significant as the population ages. For example, 92% of prostate cancer deaths occur in men over 65 years of age [14]. If projections prove correct and no mitigating interventions are developed, these numbers are going to get worse. A shift in the risk-benefit ratio of anti-cancer drugs caused by age-related decreases in tolerance plus clinical trial under-representation of this demographic worsens this picture [15]. What can be done to avert this situation?

A Potential Approach?

In 2004, one of us (Z.D.S.) proposed to the Intervention Testing Program (ITP) sponsored by the National Institute of Aging that a drug called rapamycin would mimic both diet and growth factor restriction, and, when given over a lifetime, would extend longevity. What was the rationale for such idea? Figure 1 summarizes the major stimuli that the cellular target of rapamycin (TOR) integrates in its role as a regulator of anabolic and catabolic processes. TOR, a member of a highly conserved family of stress response kinases, forms two complexes each with diverse cell autonomous and non-cell autonomous functions.

TOR research is an exploding field of studies with an average of about 40 papers reported weekly by Entrez PubMed. Although every month adds complexity to its signaling circuits (for a systems analysis, see Caron et al. [16]), the essential aspects of mechanistic (formerly mammalian [17]) TOR (mTOR) for our purposes here are illustrated in figure 1a. In addition to nutrient, energy and growth factor/cytokine

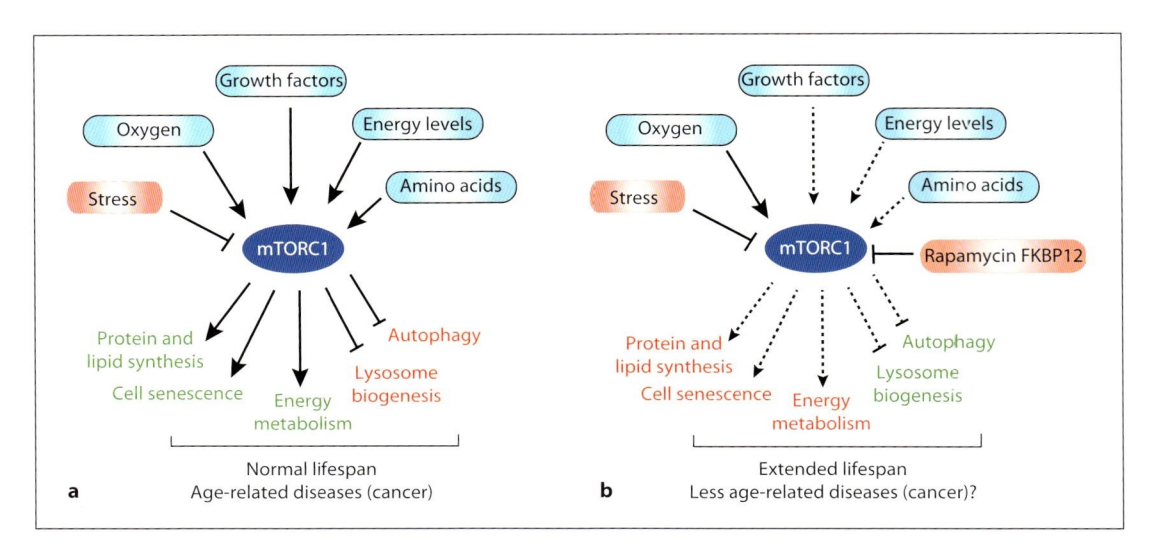

Fig. 1. mTOR complex 1 (mTORC1) signaling lifespan and cancer. **a** Major stimuli that mTORC1 integrates in the execution of its cell autonomous functions are indicated. Laplante and Sabatini [17] provided an outstanding review of mTORC1 and role in metabolism. The level of mTORC1 activity toward downstream effectors (ribosomal protein subunit 6 (rpS6), kinase 1/2 (S6K1/2), eukaryotic translation initiation factor 4E binding proteins (4E-BPs)) are indicated by the size of arrows. In a replete state (including active growth factor/cytokine upstream stimulation), mTORC1 activity is upregulated resulting a pro-anabolic (growth in mass and cell cycle progressive) state as indicated in its key outputs (red = downregulated state; green = upregulated). In adult non-proliferating tissues, activity of mTORC1 is posited to contribute to cell senescence [93, 94]. **b** Pro-longevity interventions that lead to reductions in mTORC1 activity and decrease in downstream processes. This hypothetical shift in the state of mTORC1 and the related downregulation of its key outputs is posited to result in extended longevity, including the prevention, delay and/or reduction in severity of cancer. mTOR complex 2 (mTORC2), not shown, functions in cytoskeletal organization, cell survival and metabolism [17], which in terms of aging and cancer is less well understood.

inputs, the field appears to be arriving at the conclusion that (almost) any stress placed on a cell (and thus organism) somehow impinges on mTOR to repress its activity (fig. 1). Shown in figure 1 is only one of the complexes in which the mTOR kinase participates, mTOR complex 1 (mTORC1). mTORC2 (not shown) participates in cytoskeletal organization, cell survival and metabolism [reviewed in 17]. In this chapter we focus on mTORC1 since it is currently best understood.

Also indicated in figure 1 are some of the major downstream processes that mTORC1 effects in response to diet restriction (DR), growth factor restriction and rapamycin, and which processes that are postulated to result in extended survival and fewer age-related diseases. Laplante and Sabatini [17] provided an excellent review of the role mTOR plays in the integration of growth signals, in somatic growth regulation and in diseases.

In 2005, Sharp's proposal was approved by the ITP governing body, and in 2009 *Nature* published results that tested a specially designed encapsulated formulation of rapamycin (eRapa) developed by Dr. Randy Strong (ITP Site Director at the Barshop Institute for Longevity and Aging Studies at the University of Texas Health Science Center at San Antonio) in collaboration with the Southwest Research Institute in San Antonio, Texas. eRapa is stable in food and releases rapamycin in the intestinal tract [18], and extended maximum lifespan of old (equivalent to 60 in human years) genetically heterogeneous mice of both genders [19]. A subsequent paper from the ITP showed that middle-aged mice also showed an increased maximum lifespan from chronic treatment with eRapa [20].

In this second cohort of mice, the end-of-life pathology showed that mice diagnosed with mammary, liver and lung cancer had greater mean age at death in the eRapa group. In addition, lymphoma and hemangiosarcoma as the cause of death was reduced in eRapa treated group. These data indicate that mTOR inhibition over the major portion of the life in mice pharmacologically mimics diet and/or growth factor restriction to prevent, delay and/or reduce the severity of cancer, while protecting against other age-associated diseases. Could this be applied to humans? This would depend on the biological TOR being a conserved regulator of aging and cancer.

TOR, Aging and Cancer

TOR and aging appear to have been linked during the evolution of life [21]. Although critical in development, accumulating evidence suggests that the continuation of TOR function may be dispensable, perhaps harmful, in adult somatic tissues. Reduced activity in *Saccharomyces cerevisiae* (budding yeast) [22], in adult round worms, *Caenorhabditis elegans* [23, 24], and fruit flies, *Drosophila melanogaster* [25], results in a longer lifespan. Reduced recombination of ribosomal DNA and mRNA translation, reduced acetic acid production, improved oxidative stress resistance, better mitochondrial function and improved removal of damaged proteins through autophagy are phenotypes associated with reduced activity of mTOR in yeast [reviewed in 26].

Two of the downstream signaling effectors for mTORC1 include a repressor of Cap-dependent translation called 4E-BP [27]. The other substrate for mTORC1 is ribosome subunit 6 kinase 1 (S6K1), which is thought to regulate protein synthesis via its substrate ribosomal protein subunit 6 (rpS6). Overexpression of the 4E-BP translation repressor increased longevity of *D. melanogaster* [28]. Removal of a somatic isoform of eIF4E (IFE-2), a regulatory factor for Cap-dependent translation [27], lowers global protein production resulting in an extended lifespan in *C. elegans* [29]. In addition, decreased levels of components comprising the translation initiation complex in worms (e.g., ifg-1, a homolog of mammalian eIF4G [30] and reduction of worm S6 kinase (rsk-1)) extend lifespan [31]. In an RNAi screen of *C. elegans*, Hamilton et al. [32] reported that iff-1, a homolog of the translation initiation factor eIF5A, extends lifespan. These data argue that decreased translation in worms is one mechanism for extension of survival. What about bigger organisms?

Long-lived dwarf mice also have a signaling signature in liver and skeletal muscle consistent with downregulation in mTORC1 [33, 34]. $S6K1^{-/-}$ mice have gene expression profiles similar to those of diet (calorie)-restricted (DR) mice, and females have evidence of less age-related diseases and live longer than males [35]. In sum, mTORC1 plays a major role in regulating lifespan in invertebrates and vertebrates.

Metazoan mTOR has cell autonomous and non-cell autonomous functions [36], a recent example being the regulation of intestinal stem cell renewal by extracellular signaling initiated by Paneth cells [37]. This is especially interesting in light of the finding that calorie restriction, the most robust anti-aging intervention, and rapamycin (see below) increase intestinal stem cell self-renewal via an increase in extracellular signaling (cADPR) by Paneth cells in response to a reduction of mTORC1 signaling. These non-cell autonomous functions range from the regulation of organismal growth [17] to learning and memory where it has been proposed that mTOR inhibitors may have therapeutic potential for the treatment of varied forms of cognitive deficiencies [38] and improved cognition [39]. These diverse functions make it a challenge to fully understand the precise role of mTOR in longevity regulation.

Rapamycin – A Pro-Longevity Drug That Mimics Diet Restriction – Or Does It?

Diet restriction is postulated to exert at least part of its inhibitory influence on mTORC1 through nutrient and/or energy signaling inputs (see Yilmaz et al. [37] for an example in intestinal crypt cells). A reduction in mTORC1 output also results from restricted growth factor signaling [33, 34]. Metformin indirectly inhibits mTORC1 via an inhibition of the RagGTPase system [40], which functions in the amino acid sensing system associated with lysosomes (reviewed in Laplante and Sabatini [17]). Beginning 30 years ago with phenformin, metformin and other biguanide antidiabetic drugs have been shown to extend survival in models of carcinogen-induced, genetically prone, and spontaneously arising tumors [reviewed in 41]. Would rapamycin have the same type effect?

Adding rapamycin to yeast cultures results in the cells entering a state resembling DR [42], which extends their lifespan [22]. Would this work in metazoans as a mimic of DR to increase survival? In *Drosophila melanogaster*, rapamycin treatment increased lifespan [43]. In flies whose lifespan is maximized by DR, rapamycin afforded an additional extension while it extended the shortened lifespan of overfed flies. These and other data persuaded Bjedov et al. [43] that fruit fly mTORC1 plays a major player role in age regulation, at least in fruit flies.

Previously mentioned above were our results in genetically heterogeneous mice. eRapa is the first drug formulation that extends both median and maximum lifespan in a mammal, a feat previously achieved with DR and growth factor restriction models.

Regarding cancer in these experiments, we presume that chronically eRapa-treated mice either develop neoplasms later, these neoplasms grow and progress slower (e.g., by immune protection, see below), and/or eRapa-treated mice somehow tolerate their cancers better than controls. Clearly this is an area that needs further investigation. Regardless, we can now say that a pharmacological intervention is capable of extending life leading to the question: How does it do it? And, will it improve health span (as in the case of DR)? That is, will it remove the major hurdles impeding development of the new strategies to prevent and treat cancer while mitigating the diseases associated with the gain in lifespan?

Potential Mechanisms of Rapamycin Effects on Mammalian Lifespan and Cancer

The question of whether or not chronic mTORC1 inhibition mimics DR in an aging context, and if so, the potential mechanisms (such as translation regulation and autophagy) was previously discussed [21]. Here, we focus on issues related to cancer. The high growth state (mass and proliferation) of most cancer cells is to a large degree dependent on active mTORC1 [44]. For this reason, it and its associated pathways are increasingly targeted for the development of new oncology drugs to reduce mTOR activity. Laplante and Sabatini [17] provided an excellent review of the processes (e.g., ribosome biogenesis, translation of cell cycle regulators important in proliferation, anti-apoptotic factors, angiogenic regulators, metastatic factors, and energy-promoting factors) that cancer cells exploit, and in which mTORC1 has a regulatory role.

A large body of data points to deregulated protein synthesis downstream of mTORC1 as a major requirement for cancer cell growth and proliferation. Deregulated phosphoinositide 3-kinase (PI3K) signaling pathways are frequently found in cancer. A serine/threonine kinase, Akt, is a major downstream target of PI3K [45], which is frequently hyperactive in human solid tumors and hematological tumors [46]. Eukaryotic (translation) initiation factor 4E (eIF4E) and its repressor 4E-BP have been shown to be critical players in Akt oncogenic promotion of tumor growth, while phosphorylation of rpS6 (a substrate of S6 kinase 1) appears dispensable [47, 48].

Hsieh et al. [49] recently used ribosome profiling [50] to compare the translational footprint of prostate cancer cells treated with rapamycin or ATP active-site inhibitors PP242 and clinical grade INK128 [49]. These studies revealed surprising transcript-specific control mediated by oncogenic mTORC1 signaling that included a specific set of pro-invasion and metastasis genes. These investigators also report that kinase inhibitors are more efficient in eliciting this response than rapamycin, an allosteric inhibitor. Whether these findings in prostate cancer cells are applicable to other types of cancer is a remaining question. Tumors driven by oncogenic signaling increase ribosome biogenesis linked to mTOR activation, which both of these types of inhibitors repress, suggesting that they could elicit similar responses. Will these responses be observed in tumors driven by a loss of tumor suppressor gene function? Our laboratories are currently investigating this issue.

In addition to protein synthesis, another hallmark of cancer cells is an increase in de novo lipid synthesis [17, 51, 52]. mTORC1 relays oncogenic and growth factor signaling to pro-lipogenic transcription factor SREBP1, which also promotes nucleotide biosynthesis [53]. Thus, inhibition of mTORC1 activity will likely repress these biosynthetic pathways upon which cancer cells depend.

The fact that rapamycin analogs are used therapeutically for cancer treatment (e.g., renal cell carcinoma) suggests that chronic rapamycin treatment could be beneficial in a cancer prevention setting. However, rapamycin is perceived as a potent immune suppressor, so how could it possibly be applicable to a clinical cancer prevention setting?

Tumor Immune Surveillance, mTOR and Effects of Rapamycin

Because eRapa might extend life, in part, by preventing cancer, it is worth examining how developing cancers could be eliminated before becoming clinically apparent. Tumor immune surveillance is the active process of immune detection and rapid elimination of cells that have undergone malignant degeneration. Tumor immune surveillance was initially a hypothesis of a mechanism to prevent early cancers from becoming clinically apparent, but has moved from theory to generally accepted reality.

Cancer cells express antigens that subject them to recognition and elimination by the immune system. These cancer-associated antigens are processed and presented and displayed on the cell surface with major histocompatibility complex molecules plus immune co-signaling molecules that work together to generate an effective anti-tumor immune response. Specialized antigen-presenting cells called dendritic cells are key mediators in the process of initiating anti-tumor immunity as they process and present tumor antigens to the immune cells that mediate anti-tumor immunity. Dendritic cells capture tumor antigens and use them to prime anti-tumor immunity that includes tumor antigen-specific $CD4^+$ and $CD8^+$ T cells. This tumor-specific immunity should then identify and eliminate the cancer cells. Antigen-independent (innate) immunity that can kill tumor cells includes natural killer cells and macrophages. Although this vast armamentarium of endogenous immune weapons is available for use, spontaneous rejection of clinically apparent cancers through naturally-occurring immunologically-mediated mechanisms is rare [54]. Further work in this area now makes plain that tumors employ an enormous variety of active immune escape mechanisms to evade immune elimination by host defenses [54, 55].

An important conceptual advance was the demonstration that tumor immune surveillance was the initial phase of a larger process of immunoediting [56], characterized by three E's [57]. The first 'E' is elimination of newly formed malignant cells. This phase most closely approximates what had previously been referred to as immune surveillance. The second 'E' is equilibrium. During the equilibrium phase, the continued growth of malignant cells escaping immune elimination is balanced by the evolving immune response keeping pace with the mutating tumor clones trying to escape immune elimination. The evolution of the antigens expressed by the tumor cells, and hence their antigenicity (ability to elicit an immune response) as they work to evade immune destruction is the process of immunoediting. Sufficient immunoediting eventually results in the third 'E', escape. Eventually, the evolving antigens on the tumor cells will no longer be recognized well enough by remaining antigen-specific immune cells and the tumor will grow out (escape) to become clinically apparent. Immune equilibrium has been established to occur in mouse models [58]. In humans, corroborative evidence for immunoediting has been observed in solid organ transplant recipients who all received tissues from a common donor. All got the same cancer that originated from the donors with unsuspected cancers, generally melanoma [59, 60].

Remarkably, despite the well-known fact that age is the leading risk for development of cancer and that most cancer patients are elderly (see above discussion), most preclinical evaluations of tumor immunology, including studies of tumor immunoediting and tumor immune surveillance, are done in young subjects, usually to reduce research costs associated with the study of older animals. Although anti-tumor immunity and other immune effector functions can decline with age [61, 62], the functional capacity of T cells and other immune effector arms can sometimes be therapeutically improved in aged hosts [63, 64].

Age-associated changes in immunity include reduced T cell function that could reduce anti-tumor immunity. Naive T cells in aged hosts exhibit functional defects including reduced capacity to proliferate, secrete cytokines, and undergo effector T cell differentiation [65–67]. These changes could reduce tumor immune surveillance. Nonetheless, some age-associated reductions in immune function can be reduced or reversed with specific interventions [64, 68, 69].

Chronic treatment with eRapa significantly extended the life of genetically heterogeneous mice when started at 9 [20] or 20 [19] months of age and appears to delay cancer onset [20]. mTOR inhibition has been proposed as cancer therapy largely based on its nutrient and metabolic altering properties [70]. mTOR inhibitors are approved to treat cancer or are in clinical trials. However, mTOR also has significant immune modulating properties, including effects on T cells, interferon-γ and other immune mediators critical to anti-cancer immune defenses [71–75]. Surprisingly little is known regarding how the immune modulating effects of mTOR affect cancer treatment, and nothing to our knowledge has been published regarding immune effects of mTOR inhibition in cancer delay or longevity extension.

Rapamycin is marketed as an immunosuppressive agent and carries an FDA black box warning for immunosuppression. However, rapamycin is usually used in combination with immunosuppressive agents to prevent organ allograft rejection, and thus its individual effects in humans are not well understood or studied. To our knowledge, there is no published human study of normal subjects that shows that rapamycin alone is immune suppressive. The fact that mice on chronic eRapa (achieving whole blood rapamycin levels of 10–50 ng/ml, often greatly exceeding human therapeutic levels) live longer than controls, is not consistent with any clinically relevant immune suppression. In fact, recent publications specifically looking at rapamycin immune effects demonstrate that rapamycin boosts immunity to infections [76] and is not immunosuppressive as a single agent in a mouse organ transplant model [77]. Further, rapamycin immune effects are context dependent and differ in the transplant setting versus other settings [77]. Finally, rapamycin and other mTOR inhibitors are being tested as cancer treatments in a variety of human clinical trials and are FDA-approved to treat certain cancers. It is unlikely that rapamycin would have significant anti-cancer effects if it were immunosuppressive in these populations. All available data to date suggest that single-agent rapamycin in normal hosts is not immunosuppressive, and much data supports the concept that it is an immune enhancer and beneficial to longevity as discussed and also in other settings, such as reducing coronary artery re-occlusion after balloon angioplasty in humans, and reducing Alzheimer's disease symptoms in mouse models.

In our studies of naive mice fed eRapa for 6 months starting at 6 or 19 months of age, we found no evidence for significant immune suppression, including no significant increases in immune suppressive cell populations or their function. We noted slight reductions in T cell numbers as has been reported previously, but these slight reductions were potentially offset by improvements in other factors that could augment cancer immune surveillance [manuscript in preparation]. As rapamycin has significant immune effects and can affect mediators of cancer immune surveillance, further investigations of eRapa immune effects in cancer prevention and longevity extension are warranted.

The Promise of mTOR Inhibitors in the Clinic

The first clinical use proposed for rapamycin was as an antifungal agent [78], which is its first discovered activity. Subsequent to the discovery of its anti-proliferative effects on immune cells, the FDA approved it in 1999 as an anti-rejection therapy for solid organ transplant patients. The anti-proliferative properties of rapamycin were also recognized early on making it a candidate as an antineoplastic agent. It is encouraging to find over 1,294 studies listed at the NIH site listing clinical trials (cf. ClinicalTrails.gov) using rapamycin (sirolimus (Rapamune) and its derivatives everolimus (RAD001, Affinitor), temsirolimus (CCI-779, Torisel), and ridaformalimus, formerly deforolimus). These range from small phase I and phase II trials in combination with other compounds, to large multicenter trials for advanced stage cancers. The three most common areas in which mTOR inhibitors are being evaluated for clinical use are solid organ transplantation, cancer and surgical stents with a small number in the area of vascular anomalies, infectious diseases and others. Another interesting trial planned, although not as of yet recruiting patients, is for patients with coronary artery disease over 70 years of age who will participate in cardiac rehabilitation after surgical treatment (cf. ClinicalTrials.gov identifier: NCT01649960). This trial is explicitly looking at rapamycin as a treatment for patients of advanced age.

The single most prescribed drug in the world today, metformin, was also identified as a natural compound and is also an mTOR pathway inhibitor. It is important to point out that although the molecular pathway metformin regulates primarily, the AMPK axis, has been extensively studied, we do not as of yet have a detailed systems understanding of the metformin effects in different tissue types. Nonetheless, it is a widely prescribed drug with several currently open clinical trials testing its potential use in new applications including in combination with mTOR inhibitors. Metformin is currently being assessed for murine longevity by the ITP program as well as in combination with eRapa. It will be interesting to see the results of multiple studies assessing drug responses to metformin with respect to patient age as treatment toxicities (many gastrointestinal) occur at higher frequency in this group. In addition, this patient population is much more likely to be taking other medications and have additional health issues confounding analysis. Taking metformin appears to reduce cancer risk and some recent studies link this effect directly to inhibition of the mTOR pathway [79]. It is clear that given the majority of humans requiring pharmacologic intervention are getting older on average, an emphasis on studies assessing efficacy in aged populations is essential. This argues for rapamycin as a cancer preventive given the preclinical data discussed above.

Recently developed ATP-competitive mTOR inhibitors are widely anticipated to have greater efficacy for cancer treatment [17]. The rationale for the development of this class of inhibitors was that by completely inhibiting mTORC1 and having a greater effect on mTORC2, greater efficacy could be achieved because of the strong inhibition of 4E-BP1/eIF4E and protein synthesis and more global transcriptional responses. However, like rapamycin, it is now clear that feedback loops that reactivate Akt (Thr308 [80]) could also hinder the anticipated impact of kinase inhibitors. A number of kinase inhibitors of mTOR (e.g., WYE-132, Torin1 and PP42/INK128 discussed above) and mTOR/PI3K dual kinase inhibitor (e.g., PI-103, GNE477, WJD008 and GSK2126458) have been described and tested in animal models with some having proceeded to clinical trials. However, none have been approved for clinical use to date although a number are in late-stage clinical trials.

Several reviews describe clinical uses of mTOR and mTOR/PI3K dual inhibitors in the cancer setting [e.g. 81]. They include examples in renal cancer [82, 83], bladder cancer [84], prostate cancer [85], breast cancer [86], sarcomas [86] and lymphomas [87]. A common finding is that, although mTOR inhibitors prolong progression-free survival, as a monotherapy, current drugs are not curative. From these clinical trials it appears that mTOR inhibitors are capable of boosting the anti-tumor effects of chemotherapies and in combination with other biologics such as targeted monoclonal antibody therapies have been particularly successful.

Another scenario for combining rapamycin therapy already tested involves boosting the efficacy of oncolytic virus treatment. There are a number of other preclinical models combining mTOR inhibitors with oncolytic viruses [88, 89] leading to clinical trials particularly for glioma [as recently reviewed in reference 90]. A part of this effect is clearly to reduce the clearance of virus by the immune system as is observed by using cyclophosphamide or chemotherapies; however mTOR inhibitors uniquely also sensitize tumor cells to oncoviruses in a cell autonomous manner. A genetically engineered oncolytic Sindbis virus has been found itself to be an inhibitor of the Akt/mTOR pathway late in infection cycle and holds promise as a single agent with two anti-tumor effects [91].

The co-opting of the mTOR pathway to promote viral replication and immune evasion has also been observed in studies of the herpes simplex virus and is likely not unique to these two examples. Preclinical work using vesicular stomatitis virus [92] in a rat model of malignant glioma showed rapamycin was able to increase tumor lysis at least in part by decreasing interferon production. In fact, rapamycin by itself was more effective at increasing mouse survival compared to the virus by itself and the combination extended the time to death almost three times. Interestingly, in vitro work showed that cells deficient in S6K, a target of mTOR, were more susceptible to vesicular stomatitis virus infection, consistent with the concept that boosting oncolysis is a mechanism of rapamycin action in this setting. There are a number of clinical trials combining rapamycin with immunotherapies. Bacillus Calmette-Guérin (BCG) therapy is currently standard of care in non-muscle invasive bladder cancer and is under investigation as part of a phase one clinical trial in stage IV metastatic melanoma by Dr. Alicia Terando as a phase III clinical trial at Ohio State University. Combining BCG treatment with rapamycin is an obvious next step in boosting this immunotherapeutic approach. One of us (T.J.C.) is currently conducting a clinical trial of adding rapamycin to boost BCG efficacy in bladder cancer, in conjunction with Dr. Rob Svatek here at the Cancer Therapy and Research Center.

Final Thoughts

In the cancer setting, because of the results from the eRapa ITP mouse life and health span studies described, we think rapamycin as a monotherapy has promise as a chemoprevention agent for certain cancers. Although it is premature to extend this strategy to populations with average risks of developing cancer, there are many patients with significantly increased risk of developing malignancies currently with very few options besides serial surgeries and frequent monitoring. Several investigators are also exploring clinical uses of rapamycin outside the cancer or transplantation settings. Chronic rapamycin treatment using eRapa chow greatly extends what preclinical animal experiments are feasible as it greatly facilitates administration and dosage control. We expect currently ongoing studies in non-human primates to expand our knowledge of the effects this multi-use drug where so much safety information in administration to humans is already available and well understood. Finally, it remains to be determined whether other mTOR inhibitors have superior longevity-extending or cancer prevention properties compared to rapamycin, and what specific mechanisms are involved. Understanding these issues will help facilitate clinical translation of mTOR inhibition to prevent cancer and extend life and health span.

Acknowledgements

The authors thank and acknowledge the valuable contributions of many of our colleagues whose works were not always cited in the interest of space. Supported by The Voelcker Foundation, The Hogg Trust, The Owens Foundation, The Holly Beach Public Library Association and R21 CA170491 (to T.J.C.), The Glenn Foundation (to Z.D.S.) and NIH (ISG 1RC2AG036613-01 to Z.D.S. and T.J.C.). Zachary Sharp made rhetorical improvements to the text.

References

1 Bonneux L, Barendregt JJ, Nusselder WJ, et al: Preventing fatal diseases increases healthcare costs: cause elimination life table approach. BMJ 1998; 316:26–29.
2 Juckett DA: What determines age-related disease: do we know all the right questions? Age (Dordr) 2010;32:155–160.
3 Blagosklonny MV, Campisi J: Cancer and aging: more puzzles, more promises? Cell Cycle 2008;7: 2615–2618.
4 Hursting SD, Lavigne JA, Berrigan D, et al: Calorie restriction, aging, and cancer prevention: mechanisms of action and applicability to humans. Annu Rev Med 2003;54:131–152.
5 Weindruch R, Sohal RS: Seminars in medicine of the Beth Israel Deaconess Medical Center. Caloric intake and aging. N Engl J Med 1997;337:986–994.
6 Richardson A, Heydari AR, Morgan WW, et al: Use of transgenic mice in aging research. ILAR J 1997;38:125–136.
7 Ikeno Y, Bronson RT, Hubbard GB, et al: Delayed occurrence of fatal neoplastic diseases in Ames dwarf mice: correlation to extended longevity. J Gerontol A Biol Sci Med Sci 2003;58:291–296.
8 Ikeno Y, Hubbard GB, Lee S, et al: Reduced Incidence and delayed occurrence of fatal neoplastic diseases in growth hormone receptor/binding protein knockout mice. J Gerontol A Biol Sci Med Sci 2009;64:522–229.
9 Miller RA: Geroncology: the study of aging as the study of cancer; in Esser K, Martin GM (eds): Molecular Aspects of Aging. Chichester, Wiley, 1995, pp 265–278.
10 Campisi J: Cancer and ageing: rival demons? Nat Rev Cancer 2003;3:339–349.
11 He W, Sengupta M, Velkoff V, et al: 65+ in the United States: 2005. Current Population Reports. Washington, US Government Printing Office, 2005.
12 Older Americans 2010: Key Indicators of Well-Being, Federal Interagency Forum on Aging-Related Statistics. Washington, US Government Printing Office, 2010.
13 Jemal A, Siegel R, Ward E, et al: Cancer Statistics. 2009. CA Cancer J Clin 2009;59:225–249.
14 Altekruse SF, Kosary CL, Krapcho M, et al: SEER Cancer Statistics Review 1975–2007. Bethesda, National Cancer Institute, 2010.
15 Pal SK, Katheria V, Hurria A: Evaluating the older patient with cancer: understanding frailty and the geriatric assessment. CA Cancer J Clin 2010;60: 120–132.
16 Caron E, Ghosh S, Matsuoka Y, et al: A comprehensive map of the mTOR signaling network. Mol Syst Biol 2010;6:453.
17 Laplante M, Sabatini DM: mTOR signaling in growth control and disease. Cell 2012;149:274–293.
18 Nadon NL, Strong R, Miller RA, et al: Design of aging intervention studies: the NIA interventions testing program. Age (Dordr) 2008;30:187–199.

19 Harrison DE, Strong R, Sharp ZD, et al: Rapamycin fed late in life extends lifespan in genetically heterogeneous mice. Nature 2009;460:392–395.
20 Miller RA, Harrison DE, Astle CM, et al: Rapamycin, but not resveratrol or simvastatin, extends life span of genetically heterogeneous mice. J Gerontol A Biol Sci Med Sci 2011;66:191–201.
21 Sharp ZD: Aging and TOR: interwoven in the fabric of life. Cell Mol Life Sci 2011;68:587–597.
22 Powers RW 3rd, Kaeberlein M, Caldwell SD, et al: Extension of chronological life span in yeast by decreased TOR pathway signaling. Genes Dev 2006;20:174–184.
23 Hertweck M, Gobel C, Baumeister R: C. elegans SGK-1 is the critical component in the Akt/PKB kinase complex to control stress response and life span. Dev Cell 2004;6:577–588.
24 Vellai T, Takacs-Vellai K, Zhang Y, et al: Genetics: influence of TOR kinase on lifespan in C. elegans. Nature 2003;426:620.
25 Kapahi P, Zid BM, Harper T, et al: Regulation of lifespan in Drosophila by modulation of genes in the TOR signaling pathway. Curr Biol 2004;14:885–890.
26 Kaeberlein M: Lessons on longevity from budding yeast. Nature 200;464:513–519.
27 Sonenberg N: eIF4E, the mRNA cap-binding protein: from basic discovery to translational research. Biochem Cell Biol 2008;86:178–183.
28 Zid BM, Rogers AN, Katewa SD, et al: 4E-BP extends lifespan upon dietary restriction by enhancing mitochondrial activity in Drosophila. Cell 2009; 139:149–160.
29 Syntichaki P, Troulinaki K, Tavernarakis N: eIF4E function in somatic cells modulates ageing in Caenorhabditis elegans. Nature 2007;445:922–926.
30 Sonenberg N, Hinnebusch AG: Regulation of translation initiation in eukaryotes: mechanisms and biological targets. Cell 2009;136:731–745.
31 Pan KZ, Palter JE, Rogers AN, et al: Inhibition of mRNA translation extends lifespan in Caenorhabditis elegans. Aging Cell 2007;6:111–119.
32 Hamilton B, Dong Y, Shindo M, et al: A systematic RNAi screen for longevity genes in C. elegans. Genes Dev 2005;19:1544–1555.
33 Hsieh CC, Papaconstantinou J: Akt/PKB and p38 MAPK signaling, translational initiation and longevity in Snell dwarf mouse livers. Mech Ageing Dev 2004;125:785–798.
34 Sharp ZD, Bartke A: Evidence for down-regulation of phosphoinositide 3-kinase/Akt/mammalian target of rapamycin (PI3K/Akt/mTOR)-dependent translation regulatory signaling pathways in Ames dwarf mice. J Gerontol A Biol Sci Med Sci 2005;60:293–300.

35 Selman C, Tullet JMA, Wieser D, et al: Ribosomal protein S6 kinase 1 signaling regulates mammalian life span. Science 2009;326:140–144.
36 Sharp ZD, Strong R: The role of mTOR signaling in controlling mammalian life span: what a fungicide teaches us about longevity. J Gerontol A Biol Sci Med Sci 2010;65:580–589.
37 Yilmaz OH, Katajisto P, Lamming DW, et al: mTORC1 in the Paneth cell niche couples intestinal stem-cell function to calorie intake. Nature 2012; 486:490–495.
38 Troca-Marin JA, Alves-Sampaio A, Montesinos ML: Deregulated mTOR-mediated translation in intellectual disability. Prog Neurobiol 2012;96:268–282.
39 Halloran J, Hussong S, Burbank R, et al: Chronic inhibition of mammalian target of rapamycin by rapamycin modulates cognitive and non-cognitive components of behavior throughout lifespan in mice. Neuroscience 2012;223:102–113.
40 Kalender A, Selvaraj A, Kim SY, et al: Metformin, independent of AMPK, inhibits mTORC1 in a Rag GTPase-dependent manner. Cell Metab 2010;11: 390–401.
41 Sharp Z, Richardson A: Aging and cancer: can mTOR inhibitors kill two birds with one drug? Target Oncol 2011;6:41–51.
42 Barbet NC, Schneider U, Helliwell SB, et al: TOR controls translation initiation and early G1 progression in yeast. Mol Biol Cell 1996;7:25–42.
43 Bjedov I, Toivonen JM, Kerr F, et al: mechanisms of life span extension by rapamycin in the fruit fly Drosophila melanogaster. Cell Metab 2010;11:35–46.
44 Hasty P: Rapamycin: the cure for all that ails. J Mol Cell Biol 2009;2:17–19.
45 Cantley LC: The phosphoinositide 3-kinase pathway. Science 2002;296:1655–1657.
46 Yuan TL, Cantley LC: PI3K pathway alterations in cancer: variations on a theme. Oncogene 2008;27: 5497–5510.
47 Hsieh AC, Costa M, Zollo O, et al: Genetic dissection of the oncogenic mTOR pathway reveals druggable addiction to translational control via 4EBP-eIF4E. Cancer Cell 2010;17:249–261.
48 She Q-B, Halilovic E, Ye Q, et al: 4E-BP1 is a key effector of the oncogenic activation of the AKT and ERK signaling pathways that integrates their function in tumors. Cancer Cell 2010;18:39–51.
49 Hsieh A, Liu Y, Edlind M, et al: The translational landscape of mTOR signalling steers cancer initiation and metastasis. Nature 2012;485:55–61.
50 Ingolia NT, Ghaemmaghami S, Newman JR, et al: Genome-wide analysis in vivo of translation with nucleotide resolution using ribosome profiling. Science 2009;324:218–223.

51 Bakan I, Laplante M: Connecting mTORC1 signaling to SREBP-1 activation. Curr Opin Lipidol 2012; 23:226–234.

52 Laplante M, Sabatini DM: An emerging role of mTOR in lipid biosynthesis. Curr Biol 2009;19: R1046–R1052.

53 Düvel K, Yecies JL, Menon S, et al: Activation of a metabolic gene regulatory network downstream of mTOR complex 1. Mol Cell 2010;39:171–183.

54 Zitvogel L, Tesniere A, Kroemer G: Cancer despite immunosurveillance: immunoselection and immunosubversion. Nat Rev Immunol 2006;6:715–727.

55 Curiel TJ: Regulatory T cells and treatment of cancer. Curr Opin Immunol 2008;20:241–246.

56 Schreiber RD, Old LJ, Smyth MJ: Cancer immunoediting: integrating immunity's roles in cancer suppression and promotion. Science 2011;331: 1565–1570.

57 Dunn GP, Old LJ, Schreiber RD: The three E's of cancer immunoediting. Ann Rev Immunol 2004;22: 329–360.

58 Koebel CM, Vermi W, Swann JB, et al: Adaptive immunity maintains occult cancer in an equilibrium state. Nature 2007;450:903–907.

59 Stephens JK, Everson GT, Elliott CL, et al: Fatal transfer of malignant melanoma from multiorgan donor to four allograft recipients. Transplantation 2000;70:232–236.

60 Strauss DC, Thomas JM: Transmission of donor melanoma by organ transplantation. Lancet Oncol 2010;11:790–796.

61 Fulop T, Larbi A, Kotb R, et al: Aging, immunity, and cancer. Discov Med 2011;11:537–550.

62 Vallejo AN: Immunological hurdles of ageing: indispensable research of the human model. Ageing Res Rev 2011;10:315–318.

63 Haynes L, Eaton SM, Burns EM, et al: Inflammatory cytokines overcome age-related defects in CD4 T-cell responses in vivo. J Immunol 2004;172: 5194–5199.

64 Hurez V, Daniel BJ, Sun L, et al: Mitigating age-related immune dysfunction heightens the efficacy of tumor immunotherapy in aged mice. Cancer Res 2012;72:2089–2099.

65 Rosenkranz D, Weyer S, Tolosa E, et al: Higher frequency of regulatory T cells in the elderly and increased suppressive activity in neurodegeneration. J Neuroimmunol 2007;188:117–127.

66 Ruby CE, Weinberg AD: OX40-enhanced tumor rejection and effector T cell differentiation decreases with age. J Immunol 2009;182:1481–1489.

67 Zhang H, Podojil JR, Luo X, et al: Intrinsic and induced regulation of the age-associated onset of spontaneous experimental autoimmune encephalomyelitis. J Immunol 2008;181:4638–4647.

68 Bansal-Pakala P, Croft M: Defective T cell priming associated with aging can be rescued by signaling through 4-1BB (CD137). J Immunol 2002;169: 5005–5009.

69 Lustgarten J, Dominguez AL, Thoman M: Aged mice develop protective antitumor immune responses with appropriate costimulation. J Immunol 2004; 173:4510–4515.

70 Shi Y, August DA: A new trick for an old drug: mTOR inhibitor rapamycin augments the effect of fluorouracil on hepatocellular carcinoma by inducing cell senescence. Cancer Biol Ther 2008;7: 397–398.

71 Araki K, Turner AP, Shaffer VO, et al: mTOR regulates memory CD8 T-cell differentiation. Nature 2009;460:108–112.

72 Delgoffe GM, Kole TP, Zheng Y, et al: The mTOR kinase differentially regulates effector and regulatory T cell lineage commitment. Immunity 2009;30: 832–844.

73 Haxhinasto S, Mathis D, Benoist C: The AKT-mTOR axis regulates de novo differentiation of CD4+Foxp3+ cells. J Exp Med 2008;205:565–574.

74 Weichhart T, Costantino G, Poglitsch M, et al: The TSC-mTOR signaling pathway regulates the innate inflammatory response. Immunity 2008;29:565–577.

75 Weichhart T, Saemann MD: The multiple facets of mTOR in immunity. Trends Immunol 2009;30: 218–226.

76 Vezys V, Yates A, Casey KA, et al: Memory CD8 T-cell compartment grows in size with immunological experience. Nature 2009;457:196–199.

77 Ferrer IR, Wagener ME, Robertson JM, et al: Cutting edge: rapamycin augments pathogen-specific but not graft-reactive CD8+ T cell responses. J Immunol 2010;185:2004–2008.

78 Vezina C, Kudelski A, Sehgal SN: Rapamycin (AY-22,989), a new antifungal antibiotic. I. Taxonomy of the producing streptomycete and isolation of the active principle. J Antibiot 1975;28:721–726.

79 Chaudhary SC, Kurundkar D, Elmets CA, et al: Metformin, an antidiabetic agent reduces growth of cutaneous squamous cell carcinoma by targeting mTOR signaling pathway. Photochem Photobiol 2012;88:1149–1156.

80 Peterson TR, Laplante M, Thoreen CC, et al: DEPTOR is an mTOR inhibitor frequently overexpressed in multiple myeloma cells and required for their survival. Cell 2009;137:873–886.

81 Khokhar NZ, Altman JK, Platanias LC: Emerging roles for mammalian target of rapamycin inhibitors in the treatment of solid tumors and hematological malignancies. Curr Opin Oncol 2011;23:578–586.

82 Pal SK, Figlin RA: Future directions of mammalian target of rapamycin (mTOR) inhibitor therapy in renal cell carcinoma. Target Oncol 2011;6:5–16.

83 Coppin C, Kollmannsberger C, Le L, et al: Targeted therapy for advanced renal cell cancer: a Cochrane systematic review of published randomised trials. BJU Int 2011;108:1556–1563.

84 Vishnu P, Mathew J, Tan WW: Current therapeutic strategies for invasive and metastatic bladder cancer. Onco Targets Ther 2011;4:97–113.

85 Burgio SL, Fabbri F, Seymour IJ, et al: Perspectives on mTOR inhibitors for castration-refractory prostate cancer. Current Cancer Drug Targets 2012, E-pub ahead of print.

86 O'Regan R, Hawk NN: mTOR inhibition in breast cancer: unraveling the complex mechanisms of mTOR signal transduction and its clinical implications in therapy. Expert Opin Ther Targets 2011;15:859–872.

87 Argyriou P, Economopoulou P, Papageorgiou S: The role of mTOR Inhibitors for the treatment of B-cell lymphomas. Adv Hematol 2012;2012:435342.

88 Stanford MM, Shaban M, Barrett JW, et al: Myxoma virus oncolysis of primary and metastatic B16F10 mouse tumors in vivo. Mol Ther 2008;16:52–59.

89 Lun XQ, Zhou H, Alain T, et al: Targeting human medulloblastoma: oncolytic virotherapy with myxoma virus is enhanced by rapamycin. Cancer Res 2007;67:8818–8827.

90 Perry J, Okamoto M, Guiou M, et al: Novel therapies in glioblastoma. Neurol Res Int 2012;2012:428565.

91 Mohankumar V, Dhanushkodi NR, Raju R: Sindbis virus replication, is insensitive to rapamycin and torin1, and suppresses Akt/mTOR pathway late during infection in HEK cells. Biochem Biophys Res Commun 2011;406:262–267.

92 Alain T, Lun X, Martineau Y, et al: Vesicular stomatitis virus oncolysis is potentiated by impairing mTORC1-dependent type I IFN production. Proc Natl Acad Sci USA 2010;107:1576–1581.

93 Demidenko ZN, Blagosklonny MV: Growth stimulation leads to cellular senescence when the cell cycle is blocked. Cell Cycle 2008;7:3355–3361.

94 Demidenko ZN, Zubova SG, Bukreeva EI, et al: Rapamycin decelerates cellular senescence. Cell Cycle 2009;8:1888–1895.

Zelton Dave Sharp, PhD
Department of Molecular Medicine, Institute of Biotechnology
The University of Texas Health Science Center at San Antonio
15355 Lambda Drive, San Antonio, TX 78245-3207 (USA)
E-Mail Sharp@uthscsa.edu

Senescent Cells and Their Secretory Phenotype as Targets for Cancer Therapy

Michael C. Velarde[a] · Marco Demaria[a] · Judith Campisi[a,b]

[a]Buck Institute for Research on Aging, Novato, Calif., and [b]Lawrence Berkeley National Laboratory, Berkeley, Calif., USA

Abstract

Cancer is a devastating disease that increases exponentially with age. Cancer arises from cells that proliferate in an unregulated manner, an attribute that is countered by cellular senescence. Cellular senescence is a potent tumor-suppressive process that halts the proliferation, essentially irreversibly, of cells at risk for malignant transformation. A number of anti-cancer drugs have emerged that induce tumor cells to undergo cellular senescence. However, although a senescence response can halt the proliferation of cancer cells, the presence of senescent cells in tissues has been associated with age-related diseases, including, ironically, late-life cancer. Thus, anti-cancer therapies that can induce senescence might also drive aging phenotypes and age-related pathology. The deleterious effects of senescent cells most likely derive from their senescence-associated secretory phenotype or SASP. The SASP entails the secretion of numerous inflammatory cytokines, growth factors and proteases that can render the tissue microenvironment favorable for tumor growth. Here, we discuss the beneficial and detrimental effects of inducing cellular senescence, and propose strategies for targeting senescent cells as a means to fight cancer.

Copyright © 2013 S. Karger AG, Basel

Cancer and Aging

Cancer is the second most common cause of mortality in the USA, according to a 2007 report [1]. Nonetheless, cancer death rates have declined by more than 1% per year in men and women over the past 10 years, most likely due to advances in biomedical research; still, more than 1.6 million new cancer cases and half a million deaths from cancer are projected to occur in the USA in 2012 [2]. It is notable that the yearly decline in the cancer death rate is most prominent in younger, compared to older (>45 years of age), individuals [3].

Age is the single most significant risk factor for developing cancer, and the vast majority of malignant tumors that are treated in clinics today occur in older patients

[4, 5]. Moreover, age is an important variable that promotes a pro-carcinogenic tissue environment [6]. Hence, in order to develop effective preventive and therapeutic strategies against cancer, it is crucial that we understand the relationship between aging and cancer.

Cellular Senescence during Aging

Normal human cells have a limited capacity to divide in culture [7]. This essentially irreversible loss of ability to proliferate, even in the presence of growth stimuli, is termed cellular senescence. Cellular senescence has been observed during the aging of several tissues [8, 9]. Senescent cells are linked to several age-associated tissue pathologies, such as osteoarthritis and cardiovascular diseases [10, 11]. Mutations and polymorphisms in senescence-associated genes, such as the cyclin-dependent kinase inhibitor 2A (CDKN2A) gene (p16^{INK4a} and p14/p19^{ARF}), are implicated in age-related diseases such as coronary heart disease and type 2 diabetes [12–14]. Moreover, the induction of cellular senescence by accelerating telomere shortening in mice can modulate several aspects of aging in numerous tissues and the intact organism [15]. Recently, the elimination of senescent (p16-positive) cells in a premature aging mouse model was shown to delay the progression of certain age-related phenotypes and pathologies [16].

Numerous stimuli can induce cellular senescence. These stimuli include telomere shortening [17], oncogene activation [18], DNA damage [19], activation of tumor suppressor pathways [20], oxidative stress [21, 22], and disrupted chromatin organization [23]. An accumulation of insults resulting from one or more of these stimuli during aging is thought to play a role in the etiology of age-associated degenerative and hyperplastic diseases. Identifying the signaling pathways involved in triggering cellular senescence and understanding the consequences of the accumulation of senescent cells during aging may help design therapeutic strategies to mitigate age-related pathophysiology, including age-related cancer.

Cellular Senescence and Tumor Suppression

Cellular senescence is recognized as a potent tumor-suppressive mechanism [24]. The induction of cellular senescence prevents the proliferation of potential tumor cells (cells at risk for malignant transformation) by both cell autonomous and non-cell autonomous mechanisms. The presence of senescent cells in premalignant lesions in various mouse tumor models and human patients [25, 26] is consistent with cellular senescence acting as a brake to the development of cancer. Indeed, tumor cells must bypass the mechanisms that impose cellular senescence response in order to proliferate.

Cell Autonomous Tumor Suppression

The induction and maintenance of the senescence growth arrest depend on the functions of both the Arf/p53/p21 and p16/pRb tumor suppressor pathways [26]. Upregulation of either one or both of these pathways causes an essentially permanent senescence growth arrest. These tumor suppressor pathways inhibit the expression and/or function of genes that promote cell cycle progression. Mutation or epigenetic silencing of at least one crucial regulator of these tumor suppressor pathways allows cancer cells to bypass the senescence checkpoint and progress towards tumorigenesis [18].

Non-Cell Autonomous Tumor Suppression

In addition to the permanent cell cycle arrest, senescent cells show distinct changes in gene expression [27], including microRNA expression [28], and extracellular matrix composition [29]. These changes are distinct from those that typically occur during quiescence or terminal differentiation. Cellular senescence entails a robust increase in the expression and secretion of numerous cytokines, chemokines, growth factors and proteases, which are collectively referred to as the senescence-associated secretory phenotype (SASP) or senescence messaging secretome (SMS) [30, 31].

SASP components can potentially attract and activate immune cells, which can remove nearby senescent, damaged and/or potentially tumorigenic cells [32]. Senescent cells can recruit natural killer (NK) cells and T cells to the tissue microenvironment. These immune cells can initiate cytolytic responses on senescent cells and neighboring tumor cells [33, 34]. These immune responses are important in vivo, as a recent report showed that the inactivation of NK cells by antibodies can block senescence-mediated tumor regression in a mouse model [34]. Moreover, the secretion of chemokines and cytokines by senescent cells in premalignant lesions can activate an immune-dependent clearance, termed 'senescence surveillance', by a CD4+ T-cell-mediated adaptive immune response [35].

Other SASP factors have been shown to reinforce the senescence growth arrest in an autocrine manner. These factors include the chemokine (C-X-C motif) receptor 2 (CXCR2) (also called interleukin-8 receptor 2 [IL8R2]), the protease inhibitor plasminogen activator inhibitor-1 (PAI-1), and the pleiotropic protein insulin-like growth factor binding protein-7 (IGFBP-7) [36–38].

Cellular Senescence and Tumor Promotion and Progression

Tissue microenvironments can provide a milieu that is permissive for malignant tumorigenesis [39]. Such environments are generally characterized by a sustainable supply of growth factors and a mechanism for escaping the immune system and will favor the persistence and growth of cancer cells. Interestingly, senescent cells, by virtue of the SASP, can enhance the proliferation of neoplastic epithelial cells [40]. The SASP can also promote an epithelial-to-mesenchyme transition (EMT) phenotype [41], which is a critical step in the development of metastatic cancer [42]. Further, SASP factors have been shown to promote malignant phenotypes in culture [40, 43] and tumor growth in vivo [44]. For example, senescent cells can stimulate growth and invasiveness of nearby premalignant cells in mouse xenograft models due in part to the secretion of matrix metalloproteinases by the senescent cells [45]. Hence, in ironic contrast to its tumor-suppressive action, SASP factors can also act as potent tumor promoters and thus fuel malignant tumorigenesis.

Tumor Cell Proliferation
Several SASP factors, such as GROα, IL-6 and Wnts, can be potent stimulators of cell proliferation [44, 46]. The robust secretion of these growth factors by senescent cells can stimulate and sustain the proliferation of nearby premalignant or malignant cells. Sustained tumor growth can, in turn, eventually overwhelm the host's ability to eliminate cancer cells, tipping the balance in favor tumorigenic progression. The accumulation of senescent cells with age could potentially serve as a significant source of sustaining growth factors for tumor cells. Hence, the increased risk of incurring cancer with age could in part be a consequence of the increased number of SASP-expressing senescent cells during aging. However, despite increasing circumstantial and supporting evidence, the impact of senescent cells that accumulate naturally during aging has not yet been rigorously shown to promote late-life cancer progression in vivo.

Immunosenescence and Immunoediting
A deficient or subverted immune system has also been shown to play an important role in promoting cancer [47]. While immunosurveillance eliminates damaged and tumor cells, the decreased production of immune cells during aging (immunosenescence) can reduce the ability of the body to remove tumorigenic cells, thereby promoting the development of malignant tumors. In addition to immunosenescence, the ability of tumor cells to eventually adapt to and potentially escape immunosurveillance can further favor the persistence of cancer cells. This process, often termed immunoediting, is observed in tumor cells that are continually exposed to immune cells [48, 49]. Tumor cells isolated from immunocompetent (wild-type) mice, but not tumor cells isolated from immunodeficient (e.g. RAG2$^{-/-}$) mice, were able to develop tumors when retransplanted into naive immunocompetent hosts [50]. This result suggests that tumors formed in the absence of an intact immune system are more immunogenic than tumors that arise in immunocompetent hosts. In the case of tumors that develop in immunodeficient environments, tumor cells are no longer recognized by the immune system as foreign. The presence of SASP-expressing senescent cells around tumors can potentially exacerbate tumor immunoediting and eventually permit the growth of immune-resistant cancer cells.

Cellular Senescence and Cancer Therapy

Therapies for patients with advanced cancer generally include surgical tumor resection, intensive multimodal chemotherapy, radiation therapy, or a combination of these regimens. Because the tumor-suppressive senescence growth arrest is so potent and essentially irreversible, regimens that induce tumor cells to senesce have been proposed as potential anti-cancer therapies [51]. This pro-senescence therapy approach has been developed and refined over the past few years, and currently a number of compounds with senescence-inducing activities are in clinical trials. However, the induction of cellular senescence as an anti-cancer therapy strategy is complicated by the potential pro-tumorigenic properties of senescent cells and the SASP. Thus, the ability to harness the anti-tumor activity of the senescence growth arrest must be balanced against the tumor-promoting potential of the SASP.

Senescence-Induction Therapy
Several of the widely used cancer treatments, such as certain chemotherapeutic agents, can promote cellular senescence both in culture and in vivo. Aside from their cytotoxic actions in some tumor cells, certain anti-cancer drugs, as well as ionizing radiation, can trigger cellular senescence primarily by inducing severe DNA damage [17]. The ability of these agents to promote cellular senescence could play a role in inhibiting tumor growth. Indeed, the induction of senescence in response to chemotherapy predicted a better outcome in human patients with advanced colon cancer [52]. Although many tumor cells have acquired mutations that allow them to bypass cellular senescence, reintroducing factors that can reactivate senescence pathways has the potential to repress cancer cell growth. Such factors, whether they be biological or chemical molecules that induce and/or maintain the senescence growth arrest, remain promising as therapies against cancer, provided that the potentially deleterious SASP can be blunted or ablated.

PTEN, a key mediator of the AKT/PKB pathway, is one of the most commonly lost tumor suppressor genes in human tumors, particularly in prostate cancer [53]. Loss of one copy of the PTEN gene strongly predisposes to cancer development [54], while complete PTEN loss can lead to a p53-dependent cellular senescence response [55]. For this reason, human prostate cancer does not select for complete PTEN loss, highlighting the importance of PTEN haploinsufficiency for cancer initiation and progression [56]. Therapeutic interventions that severely compromise PTEN activity or the AKT/PKB pathway can be an effective strategy to induce senescence in vivo. Importantly, PTEN-induced cellular senescence does not trigger a DNA damage response or hyperproliferative stage [57], which is typically induced by the activation of many oncogenes, and thus avoids an accumulation of damaged cells that can favor cancer progression.

Preclinical trials of pharmacological agents that activate the senescence-inducing p53/p21 pathway in cancer cells have been initiated [58]. LY83583 (6-anilino-5,8-

quinolinequinone), a pharmacological inducer of p21, can promote cellular senescence and inhibit tumor cell proliferation in cultured colorectal cancer cells [59]. Small molecules, such as PRIMA-1 and MIRA-1, which can restore the function of mutated p53, can also promote tumor regression [60, 61]. PRIMA-1^{MET} (Aprea AB) is currently in phase II clinical trials for the treatment of refractory hematological malignancies and prostate cancer. Enhancing stability and/or activity of wild-type p53 by disrupting p53/Mdm2(Hdm2) interaction has also been developed as a promising anti-cancer therapy [51, 62]. Serdemetan (JNJ-26854165), an Mdm2 inhibitor, is currently in phase I clinical trials (Johnson & Johnson Pharmaceutical Research & Development) for the treatment of advanced stage or refractory solid tumors. RO5045337, another Mdm2 inhibitor, is also in phase I clinical trial (Hoffmann-La Roche) for the treatment of hematologic neoplasms. Finally, a gene therapy approach for reintroducing p53 to fight cancer has been used in China since 2003. Gendicine™ (Shenzhen SiBiono GeneTech), an adenovirus-based vector for expressing recombinant human p53, is used as a treatment for head and neck squamous cell carcinoma.

Tumor cells are thought to be dependent on one or more specific oncogenes in order to maintain their malignant phenotypes [63]. The inactivation of a single oncoprotein (e.g. Myc) in experimental mouse tumors can induce tumor cell senescence and eventual regression of the tumors [64]. Small molecules that downregulate Myc expression or target interactions between Myc and its obligatory partners (e.g. Max) are being developed as anti-cancer therapies [65]. Quarfloxin (CX-3453), which inhibits Myc expression [66], is in phase II clinical trials (Cylene Pharmaceuticals) to treat low to intermediate grade neuroendocrine carcinomas.

Anti-SASP Therapy
While the induction of tumor cell senescence can halt tumor growth, the accompanying SASP can eventually promote the proliferation and/or invasion of neighboring cancer cells that escape the senescence therapy and/or the immune system, resulting in cancer relapse (fig. 1a). It would therefore be highly desirable to develop strategies aimed at inhibiting the cancer-promoting components of the SASP (fig. 1b). Drugs that specifically target the SASP have not yet been developed, certainly not for clinical use, but several strategies for the development of such drugs can be envisioned.

The SASP occurs as a delayed response to DNA damage [67, 68]. An important initiation event in development of the SASP is increased expression of the plasma membrane-bound form of the cytokine IL-1α, which, through a juxtacrine mechanism, activates signaling through the plasma membrane bound IL-1 receptor [69]. Thus, compounds that interrupt IL-1 receptor signaling may hold promise for preventing or suppressing the SASP.

The SASP also depends upon activation of other intracellular signaling pathways, such as the p38MAPK (p38 mitogen-activated protein kinase)/NF-κB (nuclear

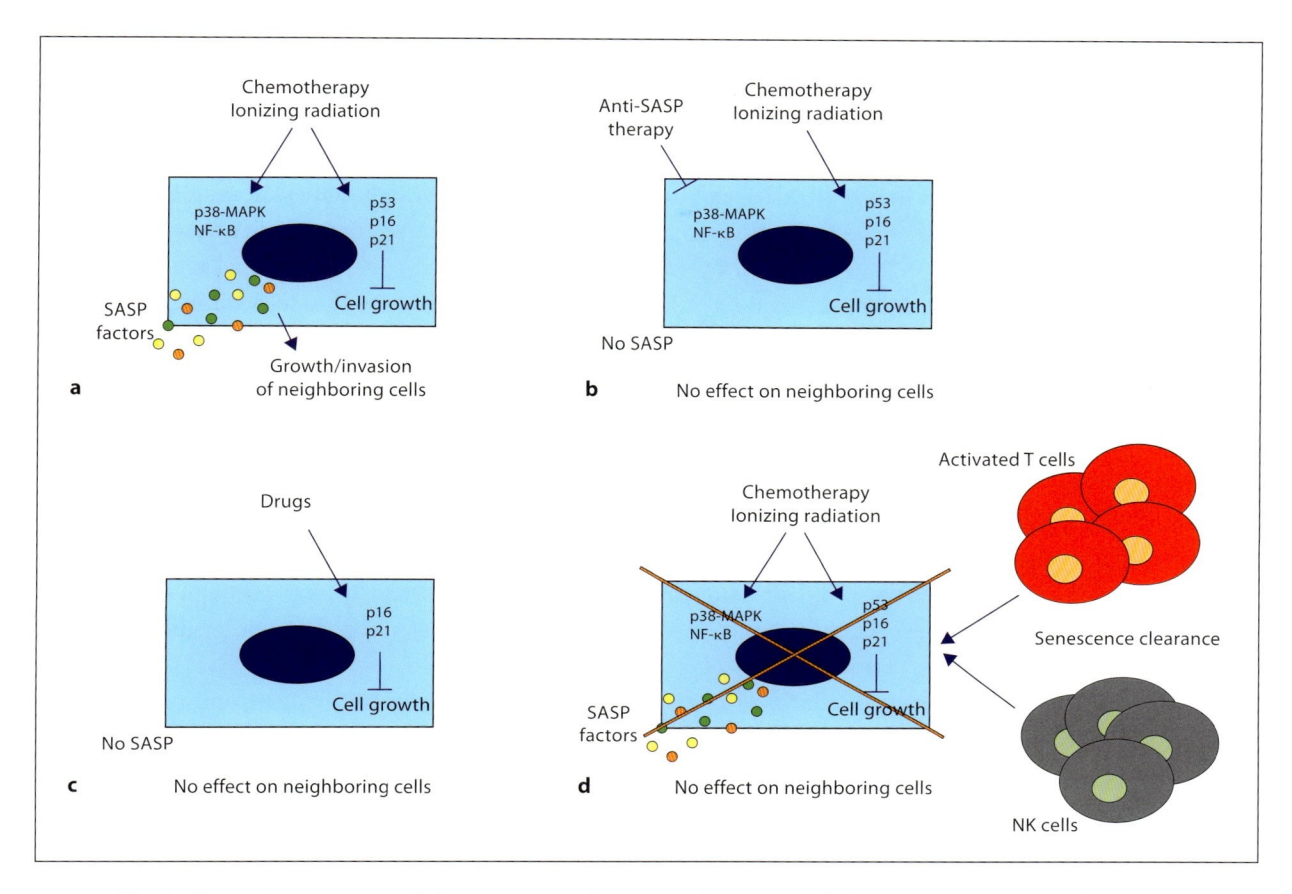

Fig. 1. Strategies to target cellular senescence for cancer therapy. **a** Cellular senescence can modulate tumor growth via cell autonomous and non-cell autonomous mechanisms. Senescent cells can express a SASP, components of which can stimulate the proliferation and/or invasiveness of neighboring tumor cells. **b** Inhibition of the SASP, or SASP components, produced by senescent cells can limit the detrimental effects of cancer therapies that induce a senescence growth arrest accompanied by a SASP. **c** Small molecules that specifically upregulate p16 and p21, without inducing DNA damage, can trigger senescence in tumors without an accompanying SASP. **d** Immunotherapy that increases immunosurveillance may help eliminate senescent cells and consequently their impact on the proliferation and/or invasion of nearby premalignant or malignant cells.

factor-κB) pathway [30, 70, 71]. Inhibition of p38MAPK is a potent repressor of the SASP, suggesting that small molecule p38MAPK inhibitors might be effective SASP suppressors in vivo [71]. Recently, as a result of a small molecule screen for SASP inhibitors, glucocorticoids (corticosterone and cortisol) were shown to inhibit the expression and secretion of several SASP factors [72]. Glucocorticoids, which are already used clinically to treat a variety of inflammatory diseases [73], may therefore be beneficial for restraining the cancer-promoting effects of the SASP.

Alternative Senescence-Based Therapy
While a SASP is observed in a variety of senescent cells in culture (fibroblasts, epithelial cells, endothelial cells, etc.) and in vivo in both mice and humans, not all senescent cells express the SASP [30, 74]. Cells that undergo senescence in response to oncogene activation, replicative exhaustion, and agents that damage DNA or disrupt the epigenome all develop a SASP. In contrast, cells that senesce owing to overexpression of the p16^{INK4a}- or p21 cell cycle inhibitors do not express the SASP [20]. One novel and potentially promising anti-cancer strategy, then, would be to develop biological or small chemical molecules that specifically upregulate p16 and p21 levels in cancer cells to induce a senescence growth arrest without inducing a SASP (fig. 1c).

Senescence-Elimination Therapy
While inhibition of the SASP following therapies that induce cellular senescence can be a potential strategy to fight cancer, the accumulation of senescent cells in aging tissues may fuel the development of late life cancer in the absence of any pro-senescence anti-cancer therapies [16]. It may therefore be beneficial to develop strategies for eliminating senescent cells, either through the immune system or through biological or chemical interventions.

Senescent cells via their SASP have been shown to attract and activate immune cells to stimulate their own clearance [33, 34]. Senescent cells express ligands for cytotoxic immune cells such as NK cells, and thus can be specifically eliminated by the immune system [33]. The accumulation of senescent cells with age raises the possibility that the aging milieu may be permissive for the retention of senescent cells. Because the immune system declines in function during aging [75], the aging immune system may also become less capable of clearing senescent cells. Thus, therapies that boost the immune system in older patients may help eliminate senescent cells (fig. 1d). The creation of antibodies that specifically recognize and trigger the elimination of senescent cells would be ideal, however such antibodies have not yet been developed.

Finally, the recent creation of a transgenic mouse model that allows the elimination of senescent cells provides proof-of-principle that the clearance of senescent cell can ameliorate the development of certain age-associated pathologies [16]. Although the effects of senescent cell clearance on the development of cancer is not yet known, this idea is now ripe for testing.

Conclusions

Aside from their cytotoxic actions, several cancer therapies that are currently in use or being tested clinically can also induce cellular senescence. While these types of therapies may prove successful in reducing tumor growth and progression, the SASP produced by senescent cells may increase the risk of cancer relapse. It is therefore important to follow the consequences of these therapies on cancer recurrence.

Inhibiting the SASP following induction of tumor cell senescence may be necessary to prevent cancer relapse. It may also be critical to develop pharmacological agents that can induce the senescence of tumor cells without triggering a SASP. In conclusion, whatever the choice of the cancer treatment, it is essential to take into consideration whether or not senescent cells are being produced, and, most importantly, whether or not these senescent cells express a SASP.

References

1. Heron M: Deaths: leading causes for 2007. Natl Vital Stat Rep 2011;59:1–95.
2. Siegel R, Naishadham D, Jemal A: Cancer statistics, 2012. CA Cancer J Clin 2012;62:10–29.
3. Heron M, et al: Deaths: final data for 2006. Natl Vital Stat Rep 2009;57:1–134.
4. Balducci L, Ershler WB: Cancer and ageing: a nexus at several levels. Nat Rev Cancer 2005;5:655–662.
5. Extermann M: Geriatric oncology: an overview of progresses and challenges. Cancer Res Treat 2010; 42:61–68.
6. McCullough KD, et al: Age-dependent induction of hepatic tumor regression by the tissue microenvironment after transplantation of neoplastically transformed rat liver epithelial cells into the liver. Cancer Res 1997;57:1807–1813.
7. Hayflick L: The limited in vitro lifetime of human diploid cell strains. Exp Cell Res 1965;37:614–636.
8. Dimri GP, et al: A biomarker that identifies senescent human cells in culture and in aging skin in vivo. Proc Natl Acad Sci USA 1995;92:9363–9367.
9. Jeyapalan JC, Sedivy JM: Cellular senescence and organismal aging. Mech Ageing Dev 2008;129: 467–474.
10. Erusalimsky JD, Kurz DJ: Cellular senescence in vivo: its relevance in ageing and cardiovascular disease. Exp Gerontol 2005;40:634–642.
11. Price JS, et al: The role of chondrocyte senescence in osteoarthritis. Aging Cell 2002;1:57–65.
12. McPherson R, et al: A common allele on chromosome 9 associated with coronary heart disease. Science 2007;316:1488–1491.
13. Scott LJ, et al: A genome-wide association study of type 2 diabetes in Finns detects multiple susceptibility variants. Science 2007;316:1341–1345.
14. Zeggini E, et al: Replication of genome-wide association signals in UK samples reveals risk loci for type 2 diabetes. Science 2007;316:1336–1341.
15. Rudolph KL, et al: Longevity, stress response, and cancer in aging telomerase-deficient mice. Cell 1999;96:701–712.
16. Baker DJ, et al: Clearance of P16^{INK4a}-positive senescent cells delays ageing-associated disorders. Nature 2011;479:232–236.
17. Shay JW, Wright WE: Role of telomeres and telomerase in cancer. Semin Cancer Biol 2011;21:349–353.
18. Serrano M, et al: Oncogenic ras provokes premature cell senescence associated with accumulation of p53 and p16^{INK4a}. Cell 1997;88:593–602.
19. Sedelnikova OA, et al: Senescing human cells and ageing mice accumulate DNA lesions with unrepairable double-strand breaks. Nat Cell Biol 2004; 6:168–170.
20. Coppe JP, et al: Tumor suppressor and aging biomarker p16^{INK4a} induces cellular senescence without the associated inflammatory secretory phenotype. J Biol Chem 2011;286:36396–36403.
21. Chen Q, et al: Oxidative DNA damage and senescence of human diploid fibroblast cells. Proc Natl Acad Sci USA 1995;92:4337–4341.
22. Velarde MC, et al: Mitochondrial oxidative stress caused by Sod2 deficiency promotes cellular senescence and aging phenotypes in the skin. Aging (Albany NY) 2012;4:3–12.
23. Prieur A, et al: p53 and p16^{INK4a} independent induction of senescence by chromatin-dependent alteration of S-phase progression. Nat Commun 2011; 2:473.
24. Campisi J: Senescent cells, tumor suppression, and organismal aging: good citizens, bad neighbors. Cell 2005;120:513–522.
25. Castro P, et al: Cellular senescence in the pathogenesis of benign prostatic hyperplasia. Prostate 2003; 55:30–38.
26. Collado M, Serrano M: Senescence in tumours: evidence from mice and humans. Nat Rev Cancer 2010;10:51–57.
27. Chang BD, et al: Effects of p21Waf1/Cip1/Sdi1 on cellular gene expression: implications for carcinogenesis, senescence, and age-related diseases. Proc Natl Acad Sci USA 2000;97:4291–4296.
28. Faraonio R, et al: A set of miRNAs participates in the cellular senescence program in human diploid fibroblasts. Cell Death Differ 2012;19:713–721.

29 Yang KE, et al: Differential expression of extracellular matrix proteins in senescent and young human fibroblasts: a comparative proteomics and microarray study. Mol Cells 2011;32:99–106.

30 Coppe JP, et al: Senescence-associated secretory phenotypes reveal cell-nonautonomous functions of oncogenic RAS and the p53 tumor suppressor. PLoS Biol 2008;6:2853–2868.

31 Kuilman T, et al: Oncogene-induced senescence relayed by an interleukin-dependent inflammatory network. Cell 2008;133:1019–1031.

32 Krizhanovsky V, et al: Implications of cellular senescence in tissue damage response, tumor suppression, and stem cell biology. Cold Spring Harb Symp Quant Biol 2008;73:513–522.

33 Krizhanovsky V, et al: Senescence of activated stellate cells limits liver fibrosis. Cell 2008;134:657–667.

34 Xue W, et al: Senescence and tumour clearance is triggered by p53 restoration in murine liver carcinomas. Nature 2007;445:656–660.

35 Kang TW, et al: Senescence surveillance of premalignant hepatocytes limits liver cancer development. Nature 2011;479:547–551.

36 Acosta JC, et al: Chemokine signaling via the CXCR2 receptor reinforces senescence. Cell 2008; 133:1006–1018.

37 Kortlever RM, Higgins PJ, Bernards R: Plasminogen activator inhibitor-1 is a critical downstream target of p53 in the induction of replicative senescence. Nat Cell Biol 2006;8:877–884.

38 Wajapeyee N, et al: Oncogenic BRAF induces senescence and apoptosis through pathways mediated by the secreted protein IGFBP7. Cell 2008;132: 363–374.

39 Liotta LA, Kohn EC: The microenvironment of the tumour-host interface. Nature 2001;411:375–379.

40 Bavik C, et al: The gene expression program of prostate fibroblast senescence modulates neoplastic epithelial cell proliferation through paracrine mechanisms. Cancer Res 2006;66:794–802.

41 Parrinello S, et al: Stromal-epithelial interactions in aging and cancer: senescent fibroblasts alter epithelial cell differentiation. J Cell Sci 2005;118: 485–496.

42 Laberge RM, et al: Epithelial-mesenchymal transition induced by senescent fibroblasts. Cancer Microenviron 2012;5:39–44.

43 Coppe JP, et al: Secretion of vascular endothelial growth factor by primary human fibroblasts at senescence. J Biol Chem 2006;281:29568–29574.

44 Krtolica A, et al: Senescent fibroblasts promote epithelial cell growth and tumorigenesis: a link between cancer and aging. Proc Natl Acad Sci USA 2001;98:12072–12077.

45 Liu D, Hornsby PJ: Senescent human fibroblasts increase the early growth of xenograft tumors via matrix metalloproteinase secretion. Cancer Res 2007;67:3117–3126.

46 Castro P, et al: Interleukin-8 expression is increased in senescent prostatic epithelial cells and promotes the development of benign prostatic hyperplasia. Prostate 2004;60:153–159.

47 Fulop T, et al: Potential role of immunosenescence in cancer development. Ann NY Acad Sci 2010; 1197:158–165.

48 Dunn GP, et al: Cancer immunoediting: from immunosurveillance to tumor escape. Nat Immunol 2002; 3:991–998.

49 Chow MT, Moller A, Smyth MJ: Inflammation and immune surveillance in cancer. Semin Cancer Biol 2012;22:23–32.

50 Shankaran V, et al: IFN-γ and lymphocytes prevent primary tumour development and shape tumour immunogenicity. Nature 2001;410:1107–1111.

51 Nardella C, et al: Pro-senescence therapy for cancer treatment. Nat Rev Cancer 2011;11:503–511.

52 Haugstetter AM, et al: Cellular senescence predicts treatment outcome in metastasised colorectal cancer. Br J Cancer 2010;103:505–509.

53 Li J, et al: PTEN, a putative protein tyrosine phosphatase gene mutated in human brain, breast, and prostate cancer. Science 1997;275:1943–1947.

54 Di Cristofano A, et al: PTEN is essential for embryonic development and tumour suppression. Nat Genet 1998;19:348–355.

55 Chen Z, et al: Crucial role of p53-dependent cellular senescence in suppression of PTEN-deficient tumorigenesis. Nature 2005;436:725–730.

56 Trotman LC, et al: PTEN dose dictates cancer progression in the prostate. PLoS Biol 2003;1:e59.

57 Alimonti A, et al: A novel type of cellular senescence that can be enhanced in mouse models and human tumor xenografts to suppress prostate tumorigenesis. J Clin Invest 2010;120:681–693.

58 Athar M, Elmets CA, Kopelovich L: Pharmacological activation of p53 in cancer cells. Curr Pharm Des 2011;17:631–639.

59 Lodygin D, Menssen A, Hermeking H: Induction of the Cdk inhibitor p21 by LY83583 inhibits tumor cell proliferation in a p53-independent manner. J Clin Invest 2002;110:1717–1727.

60 Bykov VJ, et al: Restoration of the tumor suppressor function to mutant p53 by a low-molecular-weight compound. Nat Med 2002;8:282–288.

61 Wiman KG: Pharmacological reactivation of mutant p53: from protein structure to the cancer patient. Oncogene 2010;29:4245–4252.

62 Vassilev LT: MDM2 inhibitors for cancer therapy. Trends Mol Med 2007;13:23–31.

63 Felsher DW: Oncogene addiction versus oncogene amnesia: perhaps more than just a bad habit? Cancer Res 2008;68:3081–3086.

64 Wu CH, et al: Cellular senescence is an important mechanism of tumor regression upon c-Myc inactivation. Proc Natl Acad Sci USA 2007;104: 13028–13033.

65 Larsson LG, Henriksson MA: The Yin and Yang functions of the Myc oncoprotein in cancer development and as targets for therapy. Exp Cell Res 2010;316:1429–1437.

66 Balasubramanian S, Hurley LH, Neidle S: Targeting G-quadruplexes in gene promoters: a novel anticancer strategy? Nat Rev Drug Discov 2011;10:261–275.

67 Rodier F, et al: Persistent DNA damage signalling triggers senescence-associated inflammatory cytokine secretion. Nat Cell Biol 2009;11:973–979.

68 Rodier F, et al: DNA-SCARS: distinct nuclear structures that sustain damage-induced senescence growth arrest and inflammatory cytokine secretion. J Cell Sci 2011;124:68–81.

69 Orjalo AV, et al: Cell surface-bound IL-1α is an upstream regulator of the senescence-associated IL-6/IL-8 cytokine network. Proc Natl Acad Sci USA 2009;106:17031–17036.

70 Bhaumik D, et al: MicroRNAs miR-146a/b negatively modulate the senescence-associated inflammatory mediators IL-6 and IL-8. Aging (Albany NY) 2009;1:402–411.

71 Freund A, Patil CK, Campisi J: p38MAPK is a novel DNA damage response-independent regulator of the senescence-associated secretory phenotype. EMBO J 2011;30:1536–1548.

72 Laberge RM, et al: Glucocorticoids suppress selected components of the senescence-associated secretory phenotype. Aging Cell 2012;11:569–578.

73 Bijlsma JW, et al: Low-dose glucocorticoid therapy in rheumatoid arthritis: an obligatory therapy. Ann NY Acad Sci 2010;1193:123–126.

74 Coppe JP, et al: A human-like senescence-associated secretory phenotype is conserved in mouse cells dependent on physiological oxygen. PLoS One 2010;5:e9188.

75 McElhaney JE, Effros RB: Immunosenescence: what does it mean to health outcomes in older adults? Curr Opin Immunol 2009;21:418–424.

Prof. Judith Campisi, PhD
Buck Institute for Research on Aging
8001 Redwood Blvd.
Novato, CA 94945 (USA)
E-Mail jcampisi@lbl.gov

Cancer Vaccination at Older Age

Claudia Gravekamp

Department of Microbiology and Immunology, Albert Einstein College of Medicine, Bronx, N.Y., USA

Abstract

Cancer vaccination is less effective at old than at young age, due to T cell unresponsiveness. This is caused by various age-related changes of the immune system, such as lack of naïve T cells, defects in activation pathways of T cells and antigen-presenting cells, and age-related changes in the tumor microenvironment. Natural killer, natural killer T cells, and γδT cells of the innate immune system also change with age but these responses may be more susceptible for improvement than adaptive immune responses at older age. This chapter compares various studies involving adaptive and innate immune responses in elderly and cancer patients, as well as cancer vaccination at young and old age. Finally, potential new directions in cancer vaccination at older age are discussed.

Copyright © 2013 S. Karger AG, Basel

With the current rise of the elderly population, cancer is becoming an increasingly frequent disease and cause of death. From 2010 to 2030, the total projected cancer incidence in the United States for older adults will increase by approximately 67% [1]. Indeed, metastatic cancer has surpassed heart disease as the primary cause of death in people younger than age 85 [2]. Therefore, in spite of some improvements in prevention and treatment, metastatic cancer is now the most frequent cause of death in the elderly, with co-morbid conditions complicating further treatment. When metastatic, cancer often needs aggressive, second-line treatment, for which there are few options. This is particularly challenging for frail, elderly cancer patients in which co-morbidity plays an important role. Immunotherapy may be our best and most benign option for preventing or curing metastatic cancer in such patients. Unfortunately, cancer immunotherapy is less effective at old than at young age, due to T cell unresponsiveness, especially in the tumor microenvironment (TME) [3, 4]. Various age-related changes of the immune system, such as lack of naïve T cells, defects in activation pathways of T cells and antigen-presenting cells (APC), and immune suppression in the TME contribute to T cell unresponsiveness at older age [4].

Analysis of various vaccine studies in preclinical cancer models at young and old age showed that vigorous anti-tumor responses could be obtained by tailoring vaccination to older age, but in most cases T cell responses were hardly detectable. Therefore, we questioned the feasibility of T cell activation in the TME by vaccination at older age, and whether activation of innate immune responses against cancer could be a more feasible approach since innate immune responses seems less affected by aging than adaptive immune responses. To answer these questions, we reviewed adaptive and innate immune responses in elderly and cancer patients, and compared vaccine studies in preclinical models at young and old age. These studies strongly suggest that adaptive and innate immune responses should be activated against cancer through vaccination or immunotherapy, respectively, at older age. Finally, we propose new vaccine and immunotherapeutic strategies focusing on improvement of adaptive and innate immune responses at older age, respectively.

Decreased Immune Responses in Elderly

Adaptive Immune Responses
One of the most important changes in the immune system at older age is the decline in responsiveness of T cells to new antigens. This is mainly caused by a strong decrease in the number of naïve T cells (capable of reacting to new antigens) and an increase in the number of memory T cells (capable of reacting to previously exposed antigens) at old compared to young age [5]. However, other possible causes for decreased T cell responses in aged humans and mice have also been described, such as defects in T cell receptor (TCR)/CD3-mediated phosphorylation events or aberrant regulation of tyrosine kinases associated with the TCR [6], and an age-related decrease in the αβ repertoire of the human TCR [7]. The TCR is expressed by T cells, and is required for recognition of foreign antigens in association with self-major histocompatibility complex (MHC) molecules, presented by APC to the immune system, and for subsequent activation of T cells. In addition, an age-related decrease in the expression of CD28 on the cell membrane of T cells, which provides a secondary signal for T cell activation when ligated to the B7 molecule on APC, has been reported [8]. Decreased production of interleukin (IL)-2 or interferon (IFN)γ at old compared to young age in individuals vaccinated with influenza virus or in vitro upon stimulation with influenza virus has been shown as well [9].

Innate Immune Responses
Cumulative evidence indicates that aging exerts significant effects on all cells of the innate immune system [10]. This includes natural killer (NK) cells, natural killer T (NKT) cells, γδT cells, dendritic cells (DC), macrophages, and neutrophils. NK cells are the most well-known cells of the innate immune system. NK cell function has been extensively studied in relation to aging in mice and humans. Although in

25-month-old mice NK cell number and function, such as the production of IFNγ, IL-2 of perforin, is decreased at old compared to 8-week-old mice, it has been reported that in human healthy centenarians NK cytotoxicity by activation with IL-12, IFNα, and IFNγ is well preserved, but somewhat decreased in less healthy elderly [11]. In our studies we found that the production of IFNγ by NK cells induced by vaccination with an attenuated *Listeria monocytogenes*-based vaccine was almost as good in old as in young mice [unpubl. data].

NKT cells are considered to be a member from the innate immune system because of their early response against infection and perhaps against cancer. They represent a heterogeneous T cell population that shares some functional and phenotypical characteristics with NK cells. It has been reported that the number of NKT cells increases with age [12], while their Th1 cytokines decreases with age [13]. However, liver NKT cells bearing TCRγδ are not only strongly increased in number but their functions are also well preserved in very old mice and humans [14].

γδT cells also belong to the innate immune system because of their early response against infection and perhaps against cancer. They are characterized by their ability to respond to non-processed and non-peptidic phosphoantigens in a MHC-unrestricted manner [15]. In human peripheral blood, two main populations of γδT cells have been identified based on their TCR composition. The predominant subset expresses the Vδ2 chain associated with Vγ9 and represents 70% of the circulating γδT cells in adults [15]. It has been reported that the percentage of TNFα-producing γδT cells increased with age, while the percentage of IFNγ-producing γδT cells did not alter with age [16].

DC in blood or Langerhans' cells in skin play a central role in T cell activation, but the results reported so far are variable. For instance, it has been demonstrated that blood DC from old individuals can still function as powerful APC when exposed to purified protein derivate of *Mycobacterium tuberculosis* or influenza vaccine [17, 18], while others have shown that DCs from aged individuals are more mature and have impaired ability to produce IL-12 [19], or that secretion of tumor necrosis factor (TNF)α and IL-6 significantly increased upon stimulation with lipopolysaccharide and ssRNA in DC of aged compared to young individuals [20].

Decreased Immune Responses in Cancer Patients

Adaptive Immune Responses
In cancer patients, cytotoxic T lymphocytes (CTL), recognizing tumor-associated antigens (TAA) in association with MHC molecules on the tumor cells through their TCR, and expected to destroy tumor cells when exposed simultaneously to both TAA/self-MHC complexes and co-stimulatory molecules, are often found at the site of the tumor, but have evidently been unable to destroy the tumor cells [21]. Multiple possible causes have been described for this unresponsiveness of the CTL in cancer

patients [for a review, see 3]. This includes decreased expression of MHC, TAA, or co-stimulatory molecules by tumor cells, and immune suppression induced by the primary tumors. In humans and mice, many tumors secrete lymphokines or factors that inhibit vaccine-induced T cell and NK cell responses. Examples are transforming growth factor (TGF)β, IL-6, IL-10, cyclooxygenase-2, and its products prostaglandin E_2, PD-1 ligand, or indolamine 2,3-dioxygenase.

Immune cells in the TME attracted and activated by the primary tumor such as myeloid-derived suppressor cells (MDSC) also suppress T cell and NK cell responses by the production of IL-6, IL-10, TGFβ, reactive oxygen species, inducible nitric oxide synthase or arginase [22], while tumor-associated macrophages and M2 macrophages strongly suppress T cell responses through the production of IL-6, IL-10, TGFβ in the TME [23]. Interestingly, it has been reported that the TME changes with age, i.e. it appeared that the number of MDSC increases with age, and that this contributed to the T cell unresponsiveness at older age [24]. So far, little research has been performed on MDSC and T cell unresponsiveness in relation to aging. Inducible T_{regs} also play an important role in suppression of the immune system in cancer patients, through the production of soluble factors such as IL-10 and TGFβ or through direct cell-cell contact, resulting in the inhibition of T cell and NK cell responses [25]. Moreover, evidence exists that the number of T_{regs} increases with age [26].

Innate Immune Responses
In vivo depletion of NK cells leads to a poor control of tumor growth in various cancer models, indicating the importance of NK cells in anti-tumor responses and tumor surveillance [27]. Evidence exists from mice and humans that NK cells alter with age, but that they still function at older age. However, the effect of aging on NK cells against cancer has been far less extensively studied than T cells. A few reports describe that NK cells of elderly had a lower ability to respond to IL-2, lower spontaneous cytolytic activity towards tumors than young adults [28]. However, NK cells can also be used to kill tumor cells through other pathways than perforin-mediated tumor cell destruction. For instance, a clinical trial is ongoing with bortezomib which sensitizes tumor cells for TRAIL- and FasL-mediated destruction by NK cells in cancer patients between 20 and 70 years (NCT00720785) [29]. We found NK cell responses (producing IFNγ) in vivo in old mice with metastatic breast cancer after vaccination with pcDNA3.1-Mage-b [3], or with Listeria-Mage-b [unpubl. results].

NKT cells also have anti-tumor activity in mice, including lung and hepatic cancer metastases when activated by α-galactosylceramide (αGalCer), by secreting large amounts of IFNγ and IL-4, resulting in activation of other cells of the immune system including NK cells [30, 31]. In a phase I clinical trial with αGalCer in patients with solid tumors, the effect was dependent on the high number of NKT cells present pretreatment [32]. Since the number of NKT cells increases with age, αGalCer could be a potential candidate to activate NKT cells against cancer at older age.

It has been reported that the percentage of γδT cells producing TNFα decreased in melanoma patients, but that the percentage of γδT cells producing IFNγ stayed unaltered independent of age [15]. Moreover, patients with lymphoid malignancies treated with IL-2 showed improved γδT cell responses in correlation with improved objective responses to therapy [33]. The anti-tumor effect of γδT cells was confirmed by in vitro assays showing that γδT cells recognize and kill a broad spectrum of B-cell lymphomas in vitro. The absence of effect of aging on the production of IFNγ by γδT cells and their anti-tumor effect makes γδT cells a highly attractive target for immunotherapy against cancer at older age.

Improvement of Cancer Vaccination at Old Age in Preclinical Models

More than 50% of all cancer patients are 65 years or older. The vaccine studies discussed below show that cancer vaccination is less effective at old than at young age, but that tailoring cancer vaccination to older age is feasible. Moreover, innate immune responses may also be a potential target for immunotherapy against cancer.

The research group of Provinciali [34] reported that immunization with a highly engineered mammary adenocarcinoma TS/A-IL-2, protected both young and old mice from TS/A challenge which was not possible without IL-2. CD4 and CD8 T cells were present in tumors of young but hardly detectable in tumors of old mice, while macrophages and neutrophils were detected at both ages. However, protective memory responses that could reject tumor cells upon re-challenge of tumor-free mice was only obtained in young mice. Another study by Provinciali's group [35] showed that vaccination with pCMV-neuNT against Her2/neu-expressing breast tumor cells (TUBO) completely protected young mice but only 60% of the old mice from TUBO challenge, and correlated with proliferation of spleen cells of young compared to old mice, in vitro upon re-stimulation with the Her/2 neu antigen. In a later study, Provinciali et al. [36] showed that cytotoxicity of CD8 T cells was improved at old age by improved DNA uptake using the combination of intramuscular immunization and electroporation, compared to intramuscular immunization only and that this correlated with complete rejection of TUBO cells in old mice. These results suggest a poor uptake of DNA by APC at old age, and that this could be avoided by delivering the plasmid DNA by electroporation.

The group of Lustgarten [37] also found that cancer vaccination was less effective at old than at young age. They showed that young but not old mice developed long-lasting memory responses to a pre-B-cell lymphoma (BM-185). However, inclusion of CD80 to the BM-185 cell line (BM-185-CD80) plus agonist anti-OX-40 or anti-4-1BB (receptor for co-stimulation on T cells) mAb induced equally strong long-lasting memory responses at young and old age, suggesting the involvement of T cell responses. In another study they also found that adding anti-OX40 or anti-4-1BB mAb to a DC vaccine resulted in vigorous anti-tumor responses in a syngeneic

TRAMP-C2 model at young and old age, while without anti-OX40 or anti-4-1BB, protection was significantly better in young than in old mice [38]. Moreover, immunization of young and old mice with DC-TRAMP-C2 vaccine plus anti-OX40 or anti-4-1BB mAb resulted in improved CTL responses to apoptotic TRAMP-C2 cells in vitro upon re-stimulation, compared to the same vaccination without OX40 or anti-4-1BB mAb at old age, but the CTL responses were less vigorous compared to the same immunizations at young age.

Grolleau-Julius et al. [39] showed that vaccination with a DC-OVA vaccine derived from young mice was less effective against B16-OVA melanoma tumors in old than in young mice, indicating the altered TME at older age and its effect on vaccination. The group of Zhang [24] also found that the TME was altered at old compared to young age. They demonstrated that the number of MDSC increased in the tumor environment of old compared to young mice, and that this contributed to the age-related T cell unresponsiveness.

In our laboratory, we developed a DNA vaccine of Mage-b (pcDNA3.1-Mage-b) and tested this vaccine at young and old age in two syngeneic metastatic mouse breast tumor models, 4TO7cg and 4T1, both overexpressing Mage-b in metastases and primary tumors [3]. Vaccination of both models with Mage-b was highly effective against metastases at young but not at old age, and this correlated with strong Mage-b-specific T cell responses in vitro and in vivo at young but not at old age [3]. Interestingly, we found that Mage-b vaccination activated macrophages and NK cells (producing IFNγ) in old mice [3]. In another more recent vaccine study with Mage-b delivered through a highly attenuated *L. monocytogenes*, we found a dramatic effect on the metastases in the 4T1 model at young age [40]. However, we discovered that this was not solely due to Mage-b, but rather to the direct infection and kill of tumor cells by *Listeria* [40]. Since *Listeria*-infected tumor cells highly express *Listeria* proteins, the tumor cells become a highly sensitive target for NK cells and *Listeria*-specific CTL [40]. We found that the *Listeria*-based vaccine was equally effective against metastatic breast cancer at young and old age [unpubl. results]. NK cell responses were also strongly activated by *Listeria* at young and old age, and may have contributed to the reduced growth of metastases at both ages as well.

Concluding Remarks

The main conclusion from the studies analyzed here is that the innate immune system should also be considered for testing as a potential candidate for immunotherapy at older age. This is based on the following findings. While the effect of cancer vaccination on growth of tumors and metastases could be strongly improved by tailoring the vaccine to older age, as shown in the preclinical studies analyzed here, in most cases improvement was not the result of T cell activation but rather the result of other immune cells stimulated by the vaccine. Although various functions of NK, NKT, and

Improvement of cancer vaccination at older age

Adaptive immune responses
- Generation of memory T cells at young and reactivation at old age
- Recruitment of naïve T cells by IL-7
- Activation of co-stimulatory molecules by OX40 or 1-4BB1
- Elimination or polarizing MDSC by CpG, curcumin, *Listeria*, chemotherapeutica
- Elimination of T_{regs} by Abs
- Reduction of cytokines or factors that inhibits T cell activation by curcumin

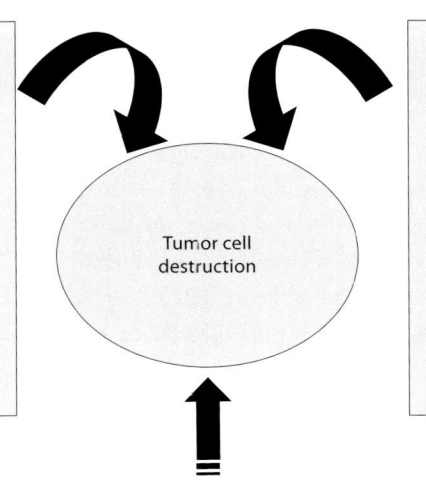

Innate immune responses
- Activation of NK cells by bacterial products
- Activation of NKT and NK cells by αGalCer
- γδT cell activation by *Listeria*
- Sensitizing tumor cells for NK cell-mediated destruction by bortezomib
- Elimination or polarizing MDSC by CpG, curcumin, *Listeria*, chemotherapeutica

Tumor cell destruction

Approaches at the tumor site
- Delivery of genes or factors into tumor cells through attenuated bacteria that leads to tumor cell destruction or improves anti-tumor responses: potential candidates are *L. monocytogenes*, or non-pathogenic bacteria such as *L. lactis* or *E. coli*
- Magnetic beads to improve delivery of compounds at the tumor site to improve anti-tumor responses or to kill tumor cells directly

Fig. 1. Various approaches to improve adaptive and innate immune responses by cancer vaccination and immunotherapy, respectively, at older age, are summarized. This includes recruitment of naïve T cells or avoid the use of naïve T cells at older age, activation of adaptive and innate immune responses at older age, by elimination of MDSC or regulatory T cells that inhibit T cell activation, activation of co-stimulatory molecules, activation of NK, NKT or γδT cells, reduction of tumor-produced factors or cytokines that inhibits T cell activation, as well as approaches that involves the selective delivery of compounds or genes in the TME that improves anti-tumor responses or kill tumor cells directly without side effects in normal tissues, such as attenuated bacteria or magnetic beads.

γδT cells are decreased at old age, it is far less dramatic than the age-related decline in T cell function, and these cells play an important role in anti-tumor responses. However, improvement of T cell activation against cancer through vaccination at older age should also be further optimized. Below, new strategies to improve adaptive and innate immune responses against cancer at older age through vaccination or immunotherapy, respectively, are proposed below and summarized in figure 1.

As mentioned above, innate immune responses should be considered as a potential target for improvement of immunotherapy against cancer at older age. For instance,

NK cells and NKT cells could be activated by attenuated *Listeria* or αGalCer, both cell types are present in sufficient numbers at older age, and both cell types exhibit anti-tumor activity. γδT cells could also be a new target for cancer immunotherapy at older age. The production of IFNγ by γδT cells seems to be unaffected by age. Moreover, patients infected with *L. monocytogenes* showed higher percentage of γδT cells than uninfected controls [41]. It has also been shown that γδT cells exhibit anti-cancer activity [33].

MDSC increases at older age and is responsible for the age-related T cell unresponsiveness in the TME. Elimination of MDSC may result in reduced immune suppression in the TME. It has been reported that CpG ODN, vitamin A, curcumin and several chemotherapeutica eliminate MDSC [42, 43]. It appears that CpG seems especially good at enhancing cellular and humoral immunity and promoting Th1-type responses in old mice [44]. We found that *Listeria* reduced the number of MDSC at young and old age [unpubl. results]. Elimination of immune suppressing tumor-associated and M2 macrophages may also lead to improved T cell activation in the TME at young and old age.

T cells could also be activated through other strategies. For instance, the problem of lack of naïve T cells, one of the most important changes at older age, could be avoided by immunizing at young age when sufficient naïve T cells are present, followed by recall at old age to reactivate memory T cells. Such an approach has been successfully used for improving antibody production at older age [45]. Also, naïve T cells could be recruited by IL-7 [46]. However, lack of naïve T cells is not the only hurdle to overcome. TAA are weakly immunogenic and T cells need help to become activated against TAA expressed by cancer cells. As shown in the studies discussed here, just adding IL-2 to TS/A tumor cells will improve anti-tumor responses but not memory responses to the tumor at old age. The best results so far have been shown by the group of Lustgarten [38] by activating T cells against cancer through vaccination plus co-stimulation using anti-OX40 or 1-4BB mAb at young and old age. Also, elimination of T_{regs} could improve T cell activation at older age [25].

Finally, we have shown that an attenuated *L. monocytogenes* can be used to deliver genes directly and selectively in tumor cells in vivo [40]. Also other non-pathogenic bacteria are currently under investigation for the delivery of genes selectively into tumor cells such as *Lactococcus lactis* and *Escherichia coli* [47]. Our results suggest that such an approach could be effective at young and old age. Also magnetic beads can be used to improve the selective delivery of agents at the tumor site that improves anti-tumor responses or kill tumor cells directly, with minor side effects on normal tissues [48].

In summary, despite all the obstacles that need to be overcome, vaccination against cancer is potentially the most promising approach. While cancer vaccination has limited success against late stage tumor development, it can be particularly effective where almost all other therapies struggle, i.e. against metastases and recurrence of cancer. The vaccine studies analyzed here show that improvement of vaccine efficacy at older age is possible, but that in addition to activation of T cells, the innate immune system should also be considered as a possible target for immunotherapy against cancer at older age. The advantage of activating adaptive immune responses by vaccination is its prophylactic and therapeutic application, while activating innate immune responses by immunotherapy can only be applied therapeutically. Finally, the results of these studies demonstrate the need of testing and tailoring cancer vaccines to older age in preclinical models before entering the clinic.

References

1 Smith BD, Smith GL, Hurria A, et al: Future of cancer incidence in the United States: burdens upon an aging, changing nation. J Clin Oncol 2009;27: 2758–2765.
2 Jemal A, Murray T, Ward E, et al: Cancer statistics. CA Cancer J Clin 2005;55:10–30.
3 Castro F, Leal B, Denny A, et al: Vaccination with Mage-b DNA induces CD8 T cell responses at young but not at old age in mice with metastatic breast cancer. Br J Cancer 2009;101:1329–1337.
4 Gravekamp C: The importance of the age factor in cancer vaccination at older age. Cancer Immunol Immunother 2009;58:1969–1977.
5 Utsuyama M, Hirokawa K, Kurashima C: Differential age change in the number of CD4+CD45RA+ and CD4+CD29+ T cell subsets in human peripheral blood. Mech Ageing Dev 1992;63:57–68.
6 Tamir A, Eisenbraun MD, Garcia GG: Age-dependent alterations in the assembly of signal transduction complexes at the site of T cell/APC interaction. J Immunol 2000;165:1243–1251.
7 Wack A, Cossarizza A, Heltai S: Age-related modifications of the human αβ T cell repertoire due to different clonal expansions in the CD4+ and CD8+ subsets. Int Immunol 1998;10:1281–1288.
8 Effros RB: Role of T lymphocyte replicative senescence in vaccine efficacy. Vaccine 2006;7:599–604.
9 McElhaney JE, Meneilly GS, Lechelt KE, Bleackley RC: Split-virus influenza vaccines: do they provide adequate immunity in the elderly? J Gerontol 1994; 4:M37–M43.
10 Gomez CR, Nomelli V, Faunce DE, Kovacs EJ: Innate immunity and aging. Exp Gerontol 2008;43: 718–728.
11 Ogata K, Yokose N, Tamura H, et al: Natural killer cells in the late decades of human life. Clin Immunol Immunopath 1997;84:269–275.
12 Mocchegiani E, Malavolta M: NK and NKT cell functions in immunosenescence. Aging Cell 2004;3: 177–184.
13 Plackett TP, Boehmer ED, Faunce DE, Kovacs EJ: Aging and innate immune cells. J Leukoc Biol 2004; 76:291–199.
14 Biron CA, Brossay L: NK cells and NKT cells in innate defense against viral infections. Curr Opin Immunol 2001;13:458–464.
15 Re F, Donnini A, Bartozzi B, et al: Circulating γδT cells in young/adult and old patients with cutaneous primary melanoma. Immun Ageing 2005;2:2.
16 Argentati K, Re F, Donnini A, et al: Numerical and functional alterations of circulating γδT lymphocytes in aged people and centenarians. J Leukoc Biol 2002;72:65–71.
17 Sauerwein-Teissl M, Schonitzer D, Grubeck-Loebenstin B: Dendritic cell responsiveness to stimulation with influenza vaccine is unimpaired in old age. Exp Gerontol 1998;33:625–631.
18 Sprecher E, Becker Y, Kraal G: Effect of aging on the epidermal dendritic cell population in C57Bl/6J mice. J Invest Dermatol 1990;94:247–253.
19 Bella D, Bierti L, Presicce P: Peripheral blood dendritic cells and monocytes are differentially regulated in the elderly. Clin Immunol 2007;122:220–228.
20 Agrawal A, Agrawal S, Cao JN: Altered innate immune functioning of dendritic cells in elderly humans: a role of phosphoinositide 3-kinase-signaling pathway. J Immunol 2007;178:6912–6922.
21 Gravekamp C, Bontenbal M, Ronteltap C: In vitro and in vivo activation of CD4+ lymphocytes by autologous tumor cells. Int J Cancer 1990;46:152–154.
22 Gabrilovich DI, Nagaraj S: Myeloid-derived suppressor cells as regulators of the immune system. Nat Rev Immunol 2009;9:162–174.
23 Sica A, Bronte V: Altered macrophage differentiation and immune dysfunction in tumor development. J Clin Invest 2007;117:1155–1166.
24 Grizzle WE, Xy X, Zhang S, et al: Age-related increase of tumor susceptibility is associated with myeloid-derived suppressor cell mediated suppression of T cell cytotoxicity in recombinant inbred BXD12 mice. Mech Ageing Dev 2007;128:672–680.

25 Shimizu J, Yamzaki S, Sakaguchi S: Induction of tumor immunity by removing CD4+CD25+ T cells: a common basis between tumor immunity and autoimmunity. J Immunol 1999;163:5211–5218.

26 Gregg R, Smith CM, Clark FJ, et al: The number of human peripheral blood CD4+CD25[high] regulatory T cells increases with age. Clin Exp Immunol 2005; 140:540–546.

27 Guerra N, Tan YX, Joncker NT, et al: NKG2D-defiecient mice are defective in tumor surveillance in models of spontaneous malignancy. Immunity 2008;28:571–580.

28 Mocikat R, Braumuller H, Gumy A: Natural killer cells activated by MHC class II targets prime dendritic cells to induce protective CD8 T cell responses. Immunity 2003;19:561–569.

29 Hallett WHD, Ames E, Motarjemi M, et al: Sensitization of tumor cells to NK cell-mediated killing by proteosome inhibition. J Immunol 2008;180:163–170.

30 Nakui M, Ohta A, Sekimoto M, et al: Potentiation of antitumor effect of NKT cell ligand α-galactosylceramide by combination with IL-12 on lung metastasis of malignant melanoma cells. Clin Exp Metastasis 2000;18:147–153.

31 Nakagawa R, Serizawa I, Motoki K, et al: Antitumor activity of α-galactosylceramide, KRN7000, in mice with melanoma B16 hepatic metastases and immunological study of tumor-infiltrating cells. Oncol Res 2000;12:51–58.

32 Giaccone G, Punt CJ, Ando Y, et al: A phase I study of natural killer T ligand α-galactosylceramide (KRN7000) in patients with solid tumors. Clin Cancer Res 2002;8:3702–3709.

33 Wilhelm M, Kunzman V, Eckstein S, et al: γδT cells for immune therapy of patients with lymphoid malignancies. Blood 2003;102:200–206.

34 Provinciali M, Argentati K, Tibaldi A: Efficacy of cancer gene therapy in aging: adenocarcinoma cells engineered to release IL-2 are rejected but do not induce tumor-specific immune memory in old mice. Gene Ther 2000;7:624–632.

35 Provinciali M, Smorlesi A, Donnini A: Low effectiveness of DNA vaccination against HER2/neu in aging. Vaccine 2003;21:843–848.

36 Provinciali M, Barucca A, Pierpaoli E, et al: In vivo electroporation restores low effectiveness of DNA vaccination against HER2/neu in aging. CII 2012; 61:363–371.

37 Lustgarten J, Dominguez AL, Thomas M: Aged mice develop protective anti-tumor responses with appropriate costimulation. J Immunol 2004;173: 4510–4515.

38 Sharma S, Domiguez AL, Lustgarten J: Aging affect the anti-tumor potential of dendritic cell vaccination, but it can be overcome by co-stimulation with anti-OX40 or anti-4-1BB. Exp Gerontol 2006;41:78–84.

39 Grolleau-Julius A, Abernathy L, Harning E, Yung RL: Mechanisms of murine dendritic cell antitumor dysfunction in aging. Cancer Immunol Immunother 2009;58:1935–1939.

40 Kim SH, Castro F, Paterson Y, Gravekamp C: High efficacy of a Listeria-based vaccine against metastatic breast cancer reveals a dual mode of action. Cancer Res 2009;69:5860–5866.

41 Jouen-Bades F, Paris E, Dieulois C, et al: In vivo and in vitro activation and expansion of γδT cells during Listeria monocytogenes infection in humans. Infect Immun 1997;65:4267–4272.

42 Lechner MG, Epstein AL: A new mechanism for blocking myeloid-derived suppressor cells by CpG. Clin Cancer Res 2011;17:1645–1648.

43 Tu SP, Jin H, Shi JD, et al: Curcumin induces the differentiation of myeloid-derived suppressor cells and inhibits their interaction with cancer cells and related tumor growth. Cancer Prev Res (Phila) 2012;5:205–215.

44 Maletto B, Ropolo A, Moron V, Pistoresi-Palencia MC: CpG-DNA stimulates cellular and humoral immunity and promotes TH1 differentiation in aged BALB/C mice. J Leukoc Biol 2002;72:447–454.

45 Stacy S, Infante AJ, Wall K: Recall immune memory: a new tool for generating late onset autoimmune myasthenia gravis. Mech Ageing Dev 2003; 124:931–940.

46 Tan JT, Dudl E, LeRoy E: IL-7 is critical for homeostatic proliferation and survival of naïve T cells. Proc Natl Acad Sci USA 2001;98:8732–8737.

47 Patyar S, Joshi R, Byrav DS, Prakash A, Medhi B, Das BK: Bacteria in cancer therapy: a novel experimental strategy. J Biomed Sci 2010;17:21.

48 Stanley SA, Gagner JE, Damanpour S, et al: Radiowave heating of iron oxide nanoparticles can regulate plasma glucose in mice. Science 2012;336: 604–608.

Assoc. Prof. Claudia Gravekamp, PhD
Department of Microbiology and Immunology
Albert Einstein College of Medicine, 1300 Morris Park Avenue
Forchheimer Bldg., Room 407A, Bronx, NY 10461 (USA)
E-Mail claudia.gravekamp@einstein.yu.edu

Immunology of Aging and Cancer Development

Tamas Fulop[a] · Anis Larbi[c] · Rami Kotb[b] · Graham Pawelec[d]

[a]Research Center on Aging and [b]Division of Haematology, Department of Medicine, Faculty of Medicine, University of Sherbrooke, Sherbrooke, Canada; [c]Singapore Immunology Network (SIgN), Biopolis, A*STAR, Singapore, and [d]Center for Medical Research, University of Tuebingen, Tuebingen, Germany

Abstract

The incidence and prevalence of most cancers increase with age. The immune system is a unique mechanism of defense against pathogens and possibly cancers, however there is a body of evidence that the immune system of the aged is eroded, a phenomenon termed immunosenescence. Each arm of the immune system, innate and adaptive, is altered with aging, contributing to increased tumorigenesis. Related to immunosenescence, a low-grade inflammation also develops with aging contributing also to increase carcinogenesis. Understanding the contribution of immunosenescence to cancer development and progression may lead to better interventions in the elderly.

Copyright © 2013 S. Karger AG, Basel

With aging the incidence and prevalence of cancer increase [1–3], which suggests a close association between aging and cancer [4, 5]. Although this relationship is not always well understood, most of the experimental data seem to sustain an essential role for time in the multihit development of cancer [1] due to accumulation of damages. Damages are induced either by free radicals or viruses rendering the oncogenes more active or the gatekeepers inactive [6]. There are well-known alterations occurring in the immune response with aging [7, 8], collectively designated as immunosenescence. However, it is still unclear to what extent immunosenescence may contribute to the development, progression and treatment of cancer in elderly subjects [9, 10]. Recently, it has been demonstrated that aging is accompanied by a low-grade inflammation, inflamm-aging, due to a disequilibrium of the immune response with aging [11, 12]. The occurrence of inflamm-aging may underline the putative contribution of immunosenescence to the increased incidence of cancer with aging.

Does the Immune System Play a Role in the Prevention of Tumorigenesis?

There are still many questions to be resolved before this question can be answered definitively. However, a variety of intrinsic tumor-suppressor mechanisms are recognized as leading to senescence and/or apoptosis to prevent the acquired capability of cells to proliferate uncontrolled [13]. It is also recognized that there are cell extrinsic tumor-suppressor mechanisms by which cancer cells are stopped from invading and spreading to other tissues. There are three major mechanisms including the limitation of specific trophic signals, the modulation of the interaction between polarity genes and proliferation, and the immune response. The immune system may play a role in tumor prevention at various levels such as eliminating the cancer-inducing viral infections, by resolving the inflammation and finally directly fighting the emerging cancer cells [14, 15]. Classically, the latter is called the immunosurveillance by which process the immune cells track modified and non-self antigens and destroy the target upon recognition. For cancer, an efficient immunosurveillance is reached when cancer cells are eliminated before formation of a clinically recognizable tumor. The immune system is controlling both tumor quantity and quality. This signifies that the immune system not only protects (quantity) against cancer formation but also influences the tumor immunogenicity (quality) [16]. Then, the concept of tumor surveillance complexified and became the cancer immunoediting hypothesis which states the dual role of the immune system toward cancer. The dynamic process of immunoediting is composed of three distinct phases: elimination, equilibrium, and escape [17]. The pre-malignant lesions appear at the stage when the immune system is able to eliminate the nascent cancer cells and this corresponds to the proper *immunosurveillance*. Mostly it consists of innate and adaptive immune responses against danger or stress signals originating from the pre-malignant lesion itself, e.g. DNA damage, apoptotic cells or the microenvironment. During the advanced oncogenesis there exists an immunoselection with an *equilibrium* status between the developing tumor and the immune system, as a consequence of the incomplete elimination of tumor cells during the previous phase. This remains still clinically unapparent. During this stage the immune system exerts a selective pressure on the evolving tumor cells and selects cells that become finally able to resist or suppress the immune response. The final stage of tumor growth corresponds to the *escape* phase where the tumor growth can be even favored by the immune system, the tumor growth [15] emerging ultimately as a clinically apparent disease. It also means that the tumor is actively suppressing the immune response by producing various inhibitory substances, e.g. NO, indoleamine-2,3-dioxygenase (IDO), PGE_2. Thus, experimental data strongly support that the immune system plays an essential role in the tumor elimination at its early stage requiring its full functionality from most of cells building the effector immune response such CD8, Th1, NK and macrophages [18]. There are several mechanisms of escape from immunosurveillance, including the alterations related to immunosenescence.

Table 1. The most important changes in the immune system with aging

Innate/adaptive immunity	Playing a specific role in carcinogenesis	
Innate immunity		
Neutrophils: decreased functions	Chemotaxis	+
	Free radical production	
	Intracellular killing	
Monocytes: decreased functions	Phagocytosis	+
Macrophages: decreased functions	Phagocytosis	
	Free radical production	
increased functions	Pro-inflammatory cytokine production	+
NK cells: decreased functions	Cytotoxicity	+
	IL-2 production	+
TLR signaling is defective on the innate immune system		+
Adaptive immunity		
Phenotypic changes	Increase of memory CD8+ T cells	+
	Decrease of naïve CD4+ T cells	
	Increase of TCR oligoclonality	
Functional changes	Decrease of clonal expansion	+
	Decrease of IL-2 production	
	Decrease in signal transduction	
Altered Th2 > Th1 balance: increased IL-10, TGF-β		+
Decrease of telomere length		
Increased T$_{reg}$ numbers		+
Increased presence of CMV seropositivity		
Low-grade inflammation		+

What Is Immunosenescence?

With aging we assist to the erosion of the immune response called immunosenescence [8, 19, 20] (table 1). This deregulation particularly affects the T cell compartment of the adaptive immune response. The most important changes in the cellular immune response with aging are (i) phenotypic, such as the decrease of naïve CD4+ and CD8+ T cells, as well as the reduced expression of CD28 with the concomitant increase of the more and more terminally differentiated memory CD4+ and CD8+ T cells characterized by surface markers such as CD95, CD45RA, CD57 and CCR7, and (ii) functional, such as a decreased proliferation, IL-2 production, telomere length with concomitantly increased DNA damage.

More and more experimental evidence shows that besides the changes in the adaptive immune response the innate immune response is also altered with aging. Each cell participating in the innate immune response is touched. Thus, natural killer cell functions are altered such as IL-2 production and cytotoxicity [21]. Phagocytic cells which are important in recognition and clearance through their Toll-like receptors (TLR) are also impaired with aging [22–24]. The functions of dendritic cells, being the main antigen-presenting cells, are also altered with aging [25].

The causes of these changes are not yet fully understood, but three main reasons can explain these changes. The first is the thymic involution with aging [26], the second are intrinsic changes because of the membrane damages leading to altered signaling [27] and thirdly the chronic antigenic stimulation occurring during life [28]. This antigenic stimulation can be of various nature – (i) from a viral source such as cytomegalovirus (CMV) of the herpes virus family, (ii) from constantly emerging tumor antigens, and (iii) from cell intrinsic sources [29]. This chronic antigenic stimulation leads with time to a low-grade inflammation characterized by the increased level of CRP, IL-6 and TNF-α [19, 30]. This low-grade age-associated inflammation was called 'inflamm-aging' by Franceschi et al. [31]. In the end, this impacts the development of age-associated chronic diseases such as atherosclerosis, diabetes, Alzheimer's disease and cancer.

Experimental evidence suggests more and more that one of the driving forces in immunosenescence is the chronic, continuous antigenic stimulation [28]. Several groups have shown an increased frequency of CD8+ T cells bearing a T cell receptor (TCR) specific for the pp65-HCMV (495-503) epitope with aging. These CD8+ T cells are highly differentiated cells from the effector memory and the effector compartment characterized by changes in their surface markers CD45RA, CCR7, CD28, and CD27. These changes in T cell phenotypes may also be induced by tumor antigens, as CD8+CD28– cells can be purified from several human tumors such as lung, colorectal [32, 33]. T cell homeostasis maintains constant numbers of T cells in the periphery and even if naïve cells continue to some extent to be generated from the thymus, the T cell repertoire will be shrunken because of the clonal expansion of these CMV-specific CD8+ T cells, contributing to increased susceptibility to infectious diseases and cancer.

These findings were confirmed in two longitudinal studies of naturally aging (>85 year) populations: the Swedish longitudinal OCTO study (donors selected for good health) and NONA (donors not selected for good health; only 9% SENIEUR-compatible (i.e. of exceptional good health) completed by Wikby's group [34, 35]. These investigations aimed at identifying factors predicting 2-, 4-, and 6-year mortality and resulted in the emerging concept of an 'immune risk profile' [36]. The immune risk profile consists of a cluster of parameters including high CD8+, low CD4+ and poor T cell proliferative response predicting higher mortality at follow-up. Other, experimental studies also suggested a special role for CMV in the loss of naïve CD8 T cells, Th1 polarization and increase of CD8+ memory T cells [37–39]. Recently, two epidemiological studies supported the data that CMV may be a primary driving force in immunosenescence by showing a correlation between CMV seropositivity, increased inflammatory markers and morbidity in elderly subjects [40, 41].

Although these experimental data clearly suggest a role for CMV, it is clear that other viruses can be implicated such as EBV [42]. Moreover, other experiments are clearly needed to understand further the effects of CMV on immunosenescence.

Furthermore, with aging we assist also to a decrease in the signal transduction of T cell surface receptors such as TCR, CD28 or cytokines. This manifests as a decrease of the phosphorylation cascade following receptor ligation, from the membrane to the nucleus (e.g. NF-κB, NFAT). Altered tyrosine kinases activation such as Lck, Fyn and adaptor molecules phosphorylation such as LAT or SLP76 at the very early stages of the receptor signal transduction are responsible for the overall reduced T cell signaling with aging [27]. These alterations originate from changes in the physicochemical properties of the membrane leading to malfunctions of lipid rafts in the membrane [43] as well as from the inability to relieve the negative signals provided by tyrosine kinases such as SHP-1.

Not only is the adaptive immune response altered, but also the innate immune response [44]. Recently it became evident that most functions of the innate immune response are affected by the aging process. Neutrophils, the first cells to arrive at the site of an aggression, have decreased chemotactic and phagocytic activities and free radical producing capacity [23]. The dendritic cells seem also to be altered not only in their basic functions such as phagocytosis, chemotaxis and production of IL-12, but also in their ability to activate naïve CD4+ T cells via antigen presentation. In the mean time they retain the capacity to produce pro-inflammatory cytokines and to activate CD8+ T cells [45]. Moreover, experimental data suggest that most of the monocyte/macrophage functions are also changed with aging, leading to altered pathogen clearing, regulation of the adaptive immune response and the inflammatory process, contributing to the sustained low-grade chronic inflammation and increased age-related diseases such as infections, cardiovascular disease and cancers. More and more experimental data indicate that with aging there are phenotypic and functional changes in NK cells, such as cytotoxicity on a per cell basis [21].

What Could Be the Link between Immunosenescence and Cancer?

We have described that aging is one of the most important risk factors for cancer. As a consequence the prevalence and incidence of cancer increases and in the mean time, immunity is compromised. There is still a debate as to whether and how the immunosenescence may contribute to this increased cancer incidence, thus the specific question that is raised: Which changes in the immune response (innate or adaptive) are responsible for the inefficient immune response against tumors?

Among the many changes in the immune response with aging are specific alterations in the innate and adaptive immune responses which contribute more specifically to the development of cancers. The immune stimulation of T cells by dendritic cells is critical for their efficient activation and this is altered in aging through the following co-receptors: B7.1, B7.2, OX40, CD27, CD30, CD40, 4-IBB [46, 47]. This leads to a weakened T cell response and even to anergy.

One important discovery of the last few years more specifically in the innate immune system is the existence of the TLR. These receptors are pattern recognition receptors (pathogen-associated molecular patterns) and can sense almost all types of antigens [48]. There are currently ten receptors which are more or less specific to various substances from bacteria, viruses or destroyed cells, which subsequently activate the innate immune system via TLR signal transduction. A wide variety of TLRs are expressed in immature or mature dendritic cells, macrophages, monocytes and neutrophils, and these receptors control the activation of these phagocytic and antigen-presenting cells [49, 50]. With aging the TLR signaling is defective in the innate immune system resulting in altered activation of the phagocytic cells which become less able to destroy the invading organisms or the transformed cells [51, 52]. Besides affecting the functions of the individual innate cells, these alterations further render neutrophils unable to activate and recruit macrophages as the next cells at the site of aggression or acute inflammation via secretion of various chemokines. In turn the cytokines released by activated macrophages should prolong the lifespan of neutrophils which is also altered with aging [53]. The described neutrophil and macrophage functional changes may as such contribute to the development and progression of tumors [23].

Aging, via the immunosenescence, favors the development and amplification of a network of immune suppressions hallmarked by increased frequency of regulatory T cells (T_{regs}: CD4+CD25+FoxP3+), myeloid-derived suppressor cells (MDSCs), IDO production, and B7 family molecules expression (B7-H1). T_{regs} maintain and induce immune cell tolerance by directly inhibiting T cells, NK cells and DCs through direct cell-cell contact [54] or by soluble mediator secretion such as IL-10, TGF-β, as well as CTLA-4 and PD-L1 expressions [55]. There is more and more evidence that the number of CD4+CD25+FoxP3+ T cells is increased in aged humans [56]. This could largely contribute to tolerance towards cancers in elderly subjects. Furthermore, MDSCs are a heterogeneous population comprised of macrophages, neutrophils and dendritic cells. They are mostly expanded in response to various soluble factors secreted by tumors such as GM-CSF, IL-1β, VEGF or PGE_2 [57]. These cells can suppress the activation of CD4+ and CD8+ T cells and inhibit the generation of antitumor responses by various mechanisms such as TGF-β secretion, TCR nitrosylation and also by the induction of T_{reg} formation and expansion [58–60]. It is of note that these cells are activated by various anti-inflammatory factors such as IL-10, TGF-β, and VEGF, which are known to increase with aging. This suggests that the increased anti-inflammatory response (Th2) or that secreted in the tumor environment favor the activation of these MDSCs which in turn can suppress the activation of an adequate immune response [61]. The IDO is an immunosuppressive molecule which is capable of inhibiting T cell activation by inhibiting CD8+ T cell proliferation and inducing CD4+ T cell apoptosis [62]. This was also shown to increase with age [63]. Thus, the increased level of IDO further contributes to the decreased immune response to tumors with aging. Finally, the B7 family molecules are involved in the regulation of T cell tolerance as well as in activation of T cell response. The accumulating data suggests that the expression of PD-L1 is altered with aging but will require further investigations to better dissect out their role in the age-related emergence of cancers.

In the adaptive arm of the immune system, alterations affect T cells, mainly naïve and cytotoxic T lymphocyte (CTL) cells with a contracted repertoire and activity shifted in favor of Th2 > Th1. This manifests in the increased production of Th2 cytokines IL-10, TGF-β, and IL-6 [61] as described above. Thus, we can summarize that the age-related specific immune alterations favor tumor development. The tumor-derived antigens are not only interacting with the professional antigen-presenting cells for activating naïve CD8 T cells but also with the CD4 T_{regs}. The naïve CD8 T cells will become cytotoxic and secrete IL-2, IFN-γ and IL-12. However, the concomitant stimulation of T_{reg} is suppressing the cytotoxic activity of CTL by producing IL-10, TGF-β and CTLA-4. Moreover, the antigen-presenting capacity of the dendritic cells is also compromised by inhibitory factors such as PGE_2, TGF-β, IL-10, and VEGF secreted by tumor cells which can induce downregulation of the number of MHC molecules [64, 65] and expansion of MDMCs. This also leads chronically to the expansion of CD8+ memory T cells which further contribute to cancer development and progression [66] by inducing DC to become tolerant to helper T cells [67]. Thus, a very tight collaboration between the innate and adaptive immune response is necessary to eliminate tumor cells. Since both arms are independently altered with aging it is obvious that this collaboration is also compromised.

It is now well appreciated that chronic inflammation can contribute to cancer development through initiation, promotion and progression [13]. Thus, one other important factor contributing to the development of cancer is the low-grade inflammation with aging [11, 12]. This arises from the overproduction of pro-inflammatory cytokines such as IL-6, TNF-α and IL-1 by the innate immune cells. This is also associated with other neuroendocrine changes such as the increased glucocorticoid or decreased IGF-1 levels. This inflammation could damage cells through the increased production of cytokines and free radicals. If so, the activation of p53 is necessary for eliminating damaged cells. However, the p53 pathway is altered with aging leading to the accumulation of damaged and possibly senescent cells which can further progress to oncogenesis [6]. As such, there is a tight connection between the immune system via the low-grade inflammation, the neuroendocrine system and the tumor-suppressor network in the organism and cells.

Moreover, as chronic antigenic stimulation plays a role in immunosenescence and the consequent low-grade inflammation, we can make the hypothesis that chronic antigenic stimulation by CMV and by cancer antigens could be additive in the induction of pro-inflammatory molecules, low-grade inflammation, and lead to more rapid immune exhaustion of the adaptive immunity and dysregulation of the immune response with aging. This in turn reduces the capacity to respond to new antigens and blunts immune responses to previously encountered antigens, including the chronic stressors. Ultimately, immunosenescence creates a favorable milieu for cancer development [68, 69].

As we have discussed, specific aspects of immunosenescence prevent an effective immune response against cancer and result in the overall increased susceptibility to cancer with aging. What the exact contribution of each parameter is still requires deep investigations. Probably there is not only one but several of them. However, if the most important parameters could be characterized the treatment offered could be more specific and efficient.

Is There an Efficient Way to Restore the Immune Response with Aging?

Experimental data support the fact that a unique therapy against cancer is inexistent [65] and there are only therapies which can be used in combination to act as multiple hits [70, 71]. The most important hits are: induction of immunogenic cancer cell death, enhancement of tumor antigen presentation, increase of gastrointestinal tract immune efficiency and blockade of the numerous immunoregulatory checkpoints.

The administration of immune adjuvants such as CD40 agonists or CpG ODNs may increase antigen presentation. The most important immunoregulatory checkpoints worthy of manipulation could be antagonists of immunosuppressive factors (e.g. VEGF, TGF-β, IL-6, IL-10, CTLA-4, IDO) and oncogenes (e.g. STAT3) and anti-apoptotic molecules (e.g. Bcl-2) and agonists to activating co-receptors (e.g. CD28, ICOS) [13]. There exist several ways to improve cancer vaccination in the elderly. Among these, the elimination of T_{reg} or macrophages suppressing T cell activation, stimulation of macrophages which can kill tumor cells, improving DC antigen presentation and recruitment of naïve T cells by IL-7 [72]. There is hope that with a better understanding of the interactions between immunosenescence and tumorigenesis, we can design better vaccines in the elderly to combat cancers.

Conclusion

The incidence and prevalence of cancers increase with aging. The aging process per se can favor the occurrence of cancers. However, the deregulated immune response also contributes. There is more and more circumstantial evidence linking immunosenescence to cancer development. However, there is no well-established study on the contribution of immunosenescence to cancer and for this reason researchers are encouraged to conduct them. A better knowledge of this interaction would help in designing better interventions. Future clinical work is urgently needed to improve the efficacy of our interventions in the growing elderly populations suffering from cancers for better treatment and quality of life.

Acknowledgements

This work was partly supported by the Canadian Institutes of Health Research (CIHR), University of Sherbrooke, and the Research Center on Aging.

References

1. Anisimov VN: Carcinogenesis and aging 20 years after: escaping horizon. Mech Ageing Dev 2009;130: 105–121.
2. Franceschi S, La Vecchia C: Cancer epidemiology in the elderly. Crit Rev Oncol Hematol 2001;39: 219–226.
3. Bürkle A, Caselli G, Franceschi C, et al: Pathophysiology of ageing, longevity and age related diseases. Immun Ageing 2007;4:4.
4. Pawelec G, Solana R: Are cancer and ageing different sides of the same coin? Conference on Cancer and Ageing. EMBO Rep 2008;9:234–238.
5. Campisi J, Yaswen P: Aging and cancer cell biology. Aging Cell 2009;8:221–225.
6. Salvioli S, Capri M, Bucci L, et al: Why do centenarians escape or postpone cancer? The role of IGF-1, inflammation and p53. Cancer Immunol Immunother 2009;58:1909–1917.
7. Fülöp T, Larbi A, Hirokawa K, et al: Immunosupportive therapies in aging. Clin Interv Aging 2007;2: 33–54.
8. Larbi A, Franceschi C, Mazzatti D, et al: Aging of the immune system as a prognostic factor for human longevity. Physiology (Bethesda) 2008;23: 64–74.
9. Malaguarnera L, Ferlito L, Di Mauro S, Imbesi RM, Scalia G, Malaguarnera M: Immunosenescence and cancer: a review. Arch Gerontol Geriatr 2001; 32:77–93.
10. Derhovanessian E, Solana R, Larbi A, Pawelec G: Immunity, ageing and cancer. Immun Ageing 2008; 5:11.
11. Miki C, Kusunoki M, Inoue Y, et al: Remodeling of the immunoinflammatory network system in elderly cancer patients: implications of inflammaging and tumor-specific hyperinflammation. Surg Today 2008;38:873–878.
12. Vasto S, Carruba G, Lio D, Colonna-Romano G, Di Bona D, Candore G, Caruso C: Inflammation, ageing and cancer. Mech Ageing Dev 2009;130:40–45.
13. Vesely MD, Kershaw MH, Schreiber RD, Smyth MJ: Natural innate and adaptive immunity to cancer. Annu Rev Immunol 2011;29:235–271.
14. Dunn GP, Bruce AT, Ikeda H, Old LJ, Schreiber RD: Cancer immunoediting: from immunosurveillance to tumor escape. Nat Immunol 2002;3:991–998.
15. Zitvogel L, Tesniere A, Kroemer G: Cancer despite immunosurveillance: immunoselection and immunosubversion. Nat Rev Immunol 2006;6:715–727.
16. Shankaran V, Ikeda H, Bruce AT, White JM, Swanson PE, Old LJ, Schreiber RD: IFNγ and lymphocytes prevent primary tumour development and shape tumour immunogenicity. Nature 2001;410: 1107–1111.
17. Swann JB, Smyth MJ: Immune surveillance of tumors. J Clin Invest 2007;117:1137–1146.
18. Poschke I, De Boniface J, Mao Y, Kiessling R: Tumor-induced changes in the phenotype of blood-derived and tumor-associated T cells of early stage breast cancer patients. Int J Cancer 2012;131:1611–1620.
19. Ostan R, Bucci L, Capri M, Salvioli S, Scurti M, Pini E, Monti D, Franceschi C: Immunosenescence and immunogenetics of human longevity. Neuroimmunomodulation 2008;15:224–240.
20. Pawelec G, Larbi A: Immunity and ageing in man: Annual Review 2006/2007. Exp Gerontol 2008;43: 34–38.
21. Gayoso I, Sanchez-Correa B, Campos C, et al: Immunosenescence of human natural killer cells. J Innate Immun 2011;3:337–343.
22. Shaw AC, Panda A, Joshi SR, et al: Dysregulation of human Toll-like receptor function in aging. Ageing Res Rev 2011;10:346–353.
23. Fortin CF, McDonald PP, Lesur O, Fülöp T Jr: Aging and neutrophils: there is still much to do. Rejuvenation Res 2008;11:873–882.
24. Gomez CR, Nomellini V, Faunce DE, Kovacs EJ: Innate immunity and aging. Exp Gerontol 2008;43: 718–728.
25. Agrawal A, Sridharan A, Prakash S, Agrawal H: Dendritic cells and aging: consequences for autoimmunity. Expert Rev Clin Immunol 2012;8:73–80.
26. Mitchell WA, Meng I, Nicholson SA, Aspinall R: Thymic output, ageing and zinc. Biogerontology 2006;7:461–470.
27. Larbi A, Dupuis G, Khalil A, et al: Differential role of lipid rafts in the functions of CD4+ and CD8+ human T lymphocytes with aging. Cell Signal 2006;18:1017–1030.
28. Pawelec G, Derhovanessian E, Larbi A, et al: Cytomegalovirus and human immunosenescence. Rev Med Virol 2009;19:47–56.

29 De Martinis M, Franceschi C, Monti D, Ginaldi L: Inflamm-ageing and lifelong antigenic load as major determinants of ageing rate and longevity. FEBS Lett 2005;579:2035–2039.
30 Gurven M, Kaplan H, Winking J, et al: Aging and inflammation in two epidemiological worlds. J Gerontol A Biol Sci Med Sci 2008;63:196–199.
31 Salvioli S, Capri M, Valensin S, et al: Inflamm-aging, cytokines and aging: state of the art, new hypotheses on the role of mitochondria and new perspectives from systems biology. Curr Pharm Des 2006;12:3161–3171.
32 Meloni F, Morosini M, Solari N, et al: Foxp3 expressing CD4+ CD25+ and CD8+CD28− T regulatory cells in the peripheral blood of patients with lung cancer and pleural mesothelioma. Hum Immunol 2006;67:1–12.
33 Ye SW, Wang Y, Valmori D, et al: Ex-vivo analysis of CD8+ T cells infiltrating colorectal tumors identifies a major effector-memory subset with low perforin content. J Clin Immunol 2006;26:447–456.
34 Wikby A, Johansson B, Olsson J, et al: Expansions of peripheral blood CD8 T-lymphocyte subpopulations and an association with cytomegalovirus seropositivity in the elderly: the Swedish NONA immune study. Exp Gerontol 2002;37:445–453.
35 Olsson J, Wikby A, Johansson B, et al: Age-related change in peripheral blood T-lymphocyte subpopulations and cytomegalovirus infection in the very old: the Swedish longitudinal OCTO immune study. Mech Ageing Dev 2000;121:187–201.
36 Derhovanessian E, Larbi A, Pawelec G: Biomarkers of human immunosenescence: impact of cytomegalovirus infection. Curr Opin Immunol 2009;21:440–445.
37 Looney RJ, Falsey A, Campbell D, et al: Role of cytomegalovirus in the T cell changes seen in elderly individuals. Clin Immunol 1999;90:213–219.
38 Chidrawar S, Khan N, Wei W, et al: Cytomegalovirus-seropositivity has a profound influence on the magnitude of major lymphoid subsets within healthy individuals. Clin Exp Immunol 2009;155:423–432.
39 Almanzar G, Schwaiger S, Jenewein B, et al: Long-term cytomegalovirus infection leads to significant changes in the composition of the CD8+ T-cell repertoire, which may be the basis for an imbalance in the cytokine production profile in elderly persons. J Virol 2005;79:3675–3683.
40 Schmaltz HN, Fried LP, Xue QL, et al: Chronic cytomegalovirus infection and inflammation are associated with prevalent frailty in community-dwelling older women. J Am Geriatr Soc 2005;53:747–754.
41 Aiello AE, Haan MN, Pierce CM, et al: Persistent infection, inflammation, and functional impairment in older Latinos. J Gerontol A Biol Sci Med Sci 2008;63:610–618.
42 Ouyang Q, Wagner WM, Voehringer D, et al: Age-associated accumulation of CMV-specific CD8+ T cells expressing the inhibitory killer cell lectin-like receptor G1 (KLRG1). Exp Gerontol 2003;38:911–920.
43 Fulop T, Dupuis G, Fortin C, et al: T cell response in aging: influence of cellular cholesterol modulation. Adv Exp Med Biol 2006;584:157–169.
44 Panda A, Arjona A, Sapey E, et al: Human innate immunosenescence: causes and consequences for immunity in old age. Trends Immunol 2009;30:325–333.
45 Agrawal A, Agrawal S, Tay J, Gupta S: Biology of dendritic cells in aging. J Clin Immunol 2008;28:14–20.
46 Morel Y, Truneh A, Sweet RW, et al: The TNF superfamily members LIGHT and CD154 (CD40 ligand) costimulate induction of dendritic cell maturation and elicit specific CTL activity. J Immunol 2001;167:2479–2486.
47 Sharma S, Dominguez AL, Lustgarten J: Aging affect the anti-tumor potential of dendritic cell vaccination, but it can be overcome by co-stimulation with anti-OX40 or anti-4-1BB. Exp Gerontol 2006;41:78–84.
48 Takeda K, Kaisho T, Akira S: Toll-like receptors. Annu Rev Immunol 2003;21:335–376.
49 Blander JM: Phagocytosis and antigen presentation: a partnership initiated by Toll-like receptors. Ann Rheum Dis 2008;67(suppl 3):44–49.
50 Wolska A, Lech-Marańda E, Robak T: Toll-like receptors and their role in carcinogenesis and anti-tumor treatment. Cell Mol Biol Lett 2009;14:248–272.
51 Van Duin D, Shaw AC: Toll-like receptors in older adults. J Am Geriatr Soc 2007;55:1438–1444.
52 Fulop T, Larbi A, Douziech N, et al: Signal transduction and functional changes in neutrophils with aging. Aging Cell 2004;3:217–226.
53 Fülöp T Jr, Fouquet C, Allaire P, et al: Changes in apoptosis of human polymorphonuclear granulocytes with aging. Mech Ageing Dev 1997;96:15–34.
54 Sakaguchi S, Yamaguchi T, Nomura T, Ono M: Regulatory T cells and immune tolerance. Cell 2008;133:775–787.
55 Terabe M, Berzofsky JA: Immunoregulatory T cells in tumor immunity. Curr Opin Immunol 2004;16:157–162.
56 Gregg R, Smith CM, Clark FJ, et al: The number of human peripheral blood CD4+ CD25^{high} regulatory T cells increases with age. Clin Exp Immunol 2005;140:540–546.
57 Gabrilovich DI, Nagaraj S: Myeloid-derived suppressor cells as regulators of the immune system. Nat Rev Immunol 2009;9:162–174.
58 Nagaraj S, Gabrilovich DI: Tumor escape mechanism governed by myeloid-derived suppressor cells. Cancer Res 2006;68:2561–2563.

59 Li H, Han Y, Guo Q, Zhang M, Cao X: Cancer-expanded myeloid-derived suppressor cells induce anergy of NK cells through membrane-bound TGF-β_1. J Immunol 2009;182:240–249.

60 Srivastava MK, Sinha P, Clements VK, et al: Myeloid-derived suppressor cells inhibit T-cell activation by depleting cystine and cysteine. Cancer Res 2010;70:68–77.

61 Huang H, Patel DD, Manton KG: The immune system in aging: roles of cytokines, T cells and NK cells. Front Biosci 2005;10:192–215.

62 Uyttenhove C, Pilotte L, Théate I, et al: Evidence for a tumoral immune resistance mechanism based on tryptophan degradation by indoleamine 2,3-dioxygenase. Nat Med 2003;9:1269–1274.

63 Pertovaara M, Hasan T, Raitala A, et al: Indoleamine 2,3-dioxygenase activity is increased in patients with systemic lupus erythematosus and predicts disease activation in the sunny season. Clin Exp Immunol 2007;150:274–278.

64 Lustgarten J: Cancer, aging and immunotherapy: lessons learned from animal models. Cancer Immunol Immunother 2009;58:1979–1989.

65 Pawelec G, Lustgarten J, Ruby C, Gravekamp C: Impact of aging on cancer immunity and immunotherapy. Cancer Immunol Immunother 2009;58:1723–1724.

66 Dock JN, Effros RB: Role of CD8 T cell replicative senescence in human aging and in HIV-mediated immunosenescence. Aging Dis 2011;2:382–397.

67 Cortesini R, LeMaoult J, Ciubotariu R, Cortesini NS: CD8+CD28- T suppressor cells and the induction of antigen-specific, antigen-presenting cell-mediated suppression of Th reactivity. Immunol Rev 2001;182:201–206.

68 Fulop T, Larbi A, Kotb R, de Angelis F, Pawelec G: Aging, immunity, and cancer. Discov Med 2011;11:537–550.

69 Fulop T, Kotb R, Fortin CF, Pawelec G, de Angelis F, Larbi A: Potential role of immunosenescence in cancer development. Ann NY Acad Sci 2010;1197:158–165.

70 Gravekamp C: The importance of the age factor in cancer vaccination at older age. Cancer Immunol Immunother 2009;58:1969–1977.

71 Gravekamp C, Kim SH, Castro F: Cancer vaccination: manipulation of immune responses at old age. Mech Ageing Dev 2009;130:67–75.

72 Provinciali M: Immunosenescence and cancer vaccines. Cancer Immunol Immunother 2009;58:1959–1967.

Tamas Fulop, MD, PhD
Research Center on Aging, University of Sherbrooke
1036, rue Belvédère Sud
Sherbrooke, QC J1H 4C4 (Canada)
E-Mail tamas.fulop@usherbrooke.ca

Metabolic Syndrome and Cancer: From Bedside to Bench and Back

Martine Extermann

Senior Adult Oncology Program, H. Lee Moffitt Cancer Center and Research Institute, University of South Florida, Tampa, Fla., USA

Abstract

As older patients present with an average of three comorbidities beside their cancer, geriatric oncology can provide unique clues to translational research in aging and cancer. We illustrate this approach with the example of the metabolic syndrome and cancer. Epidemiologic and clinical cohorts highlighted an association between the metabolic syndrome and a higher risk and worse prognosis of various cancers. In a bedside-to-bench transition, this led to an interest in analyzing the potential mechanisms underlying this association. At least ten potential mechanisms could be implicated, with the challenge of understanding which are the dominant ones in human patients. Bench-to-bedside studies are beginning to shed some light on that aspect, and some therapeutic trials are beginning to exploit the lessons learned.

Copyright © 2013 S. Karger AG, Basel

Translational research is a bidirectional endeavor and often merges knowledge from several disciplines. An excellent illustrative example is the interaction between metabolic syndrome and cancer. Such a topic is highly relevant to geriatrics, as the prevalence of metabolic syndrome increases with age to reach about 40% of the population aged 60 and older [1]. It also illustrates an increasingly recognized phenomenon: the impact of comorbidity on cancer risk and prognosis. Here again, this example illustrates the principle that a patient's diseases cannot be considered in isolation and need to be addressed in an integrated manner.

Research about metabolic syndrome and cancer started from the observation that patients with diabetes had a higher risk of cancer [2, 3] and a worse prognosis [4–9] once diagnosed. The observation was extended to the metabolic syndrome. Associations were found for example with the risk of brain [10], breast (in postmenopausal women) [11], cervical [12], colorectal [13–16], liver [17, 18], lung, pancreatic [19, 20], and prostate cancer [21], and the prognosis of breast [22], colorectal [23, 24], and prostate cancer [25, 26]. Although these associations were first described in

Table 1. Potential mechanisms by which metabolic syndrome interacts with the behavior of cancer

Insulin-like growth factor-1 pathway activation
Hyperinsulinemia/insulin resistance
Hyperglycemia, advanced glycation end-products and their receptor (RAGE)
Atypical PKC dysregulation
Leptin and adiponectin
Vascular damage and VEGF increases
Inflammation
Impaired immunity
Peroxisome proliferator-activated receptor modulation

---

middle-aged patients, they also apply to elderly patients [27]. However, epidemiologic studies provide mixed results as to which components of the metabolic syndrome matter most (insulin resistance, hypertension, hypercholesterolemia/hyperlipidemia, or obesity) [10, 12–15, 19–21, 24, 28]. Therefore, going from bedside to bench might provide some clues as to the potential mechanisms involved (table 1).

From Bedside to Bench

Several mechanisms can be postulated for the association of metabolic syndrome and cancer. They may affect the tumor, the host, or both.

(1) The most explored pathway is the *insulin-like growth factor-1 (IGF-1) pathway*. This pathway consists of IGF-1, IGF-2, several binding proteins, and the IGF-1 receptor. This receptor in turn activates the PI3K-Akt pathway and its subsequent consequences in cell growth and apoptosis. This pathway is of interest in insulin resistance syndromes because of the interactions with the insulin pathway. Insulin has some cross-activating effect on the IGF-1 receptor. The insulin-receptor and the IGF-1 receptor can also form heterodimers. This receptor is overexpressed in more than 90% of colon cancer cells [29, 30]. Its level of expression is associated with tumor grade and stage and it induces resistance to apoptosis in colon cancer cells through the Akt/Bcl-xL pathway, as demonstrated by some Moffitt work [29, 31]. Its blockade inhibits growth and angiogenesis in colon cancer [32]. Elevated plasma insulin levels activate insulin, and possibly IGF-1, receptors, and insulin itself might stimulate the IGF-1R [33]. The activity of plasma IGF-1 is modulated by its binding to IGF-binding proteins. Total IGF-1 levels and IGFBP levels decrease with age [34, 35]. However, free IGF-1 levels were found increased in subjects above the age of 70 [35]. Elderly patients may also have a small rise in the number of IGF type 1 receptors per cell [36]. IGF-1 decreases with higher BMI [34]. IGF-1 and IGFBP-1 appear to be both decreased in metabolic syndrome patients (no data on the resulting impact on free IGF-1) [37]. Diabetic patients also have decreased IGF-1 levels, correlated with poor

glycemic control and a worse outcome of cardiovascular disease [38]. No data on free IGF-1 in metabolic syndrome or diabetes are to our knowledge available, but some indirect evidence suggests it might be elevated [39]. These results point toward a somewhat complex but potentially important implication of the IGF-1/IGF-1R pathway in cancer patients with metabolic syndrome.

(2) *Hyperinsulinemia and insulin resistance.* Hyperinsulinemia might by itself activate cell multiplication. This finding is consistent with the increasing body of literature suggesting that hyperinsulinemia seems to be the critical factor in the association of metabolic syndrome and colon cancer. Increased risk of colon cancer or excess of colon cancer deaths were found in patients with recently diagnosed diabetes or impaired glucose tolerance [40]. C-peptide concentrations, which are a measure of insulin secretion, were found to be a stronger predictor of colorectal cancer risk than was the metabolic syndrome [41]. Postprandial insulin [42] and nonfasting C-peptide [41, 43], a measure of hyperinsulinemia rather than insulin resistance, are stronger predictors of colon cancer risk than is the fasting insulin concentration [42, 44]. Finally, in one study, chronic insulin therapy was associated with a significantly increased risk of colorectal cancer among patients with type 2 diabetes [45]. In addition to the epidemiologic evidence, mechanistic studies have also suggested direct mitogenic and proliferative effects of insulin on tumors [46]. Insulin has two receptors: IR-A and IR-B. The first one mediates the mitogenic effects and the second one the metabolic effects of insulin. IR-A can be aberrantly expressed in tumor cells, and has a high affinity for IGF-2 as well [47]. These receptors can dimerize with the IGF-1 receptor. It is also interesting to note that peritumoral vessels express a high level of insulin receptors [48]. Another way hyperinsulinemia might stimulate cancer growth is through the NF-κB pathway, as IKK-β appears to be a key mediator in insulin resistance. High-dose salicylates, which inhibit IKK-β, can reverse hyperglycemia, hyperinsulinemia and dyslipidemia in obese rodents in a COX-independent fashion [49].

(3) *Hyperglycemia and advanced glycation end-products (AGEs).* Sustained hyperglycemia by itself might favor cancer growth. Most tumors are glucose-avid, as demonstrated by the diagnostic effectiveness of PET scanning. This may be true for example if protein kinase C (PKC)-ζ is not turned down in tumors from metabolic syndrome patients (see below). Oral antidiabetics such as phenformin, buformin, and diabenol have been shown to inhibit colon carcinogenesis and shift phenotype to more differentiated tumors in rats [50]. Their postulated mechanism of action is a calorie restriction-like action, decreasing hyperinsulinemia, hyperglycemia, and oxidative stress. This effect may be mediated by the restoration of PKC-ζ function in the muscle. Another potential mechanism of action by hyperglycemia is AGEs. These increase with age and diabetes [51] and induce similar 'aging' changes. AGEs are produced by nonenzymatic glycation of proteins with reducing sugars and subsequent metal-catalyzed oxidations. Oxidation of glycated proteins or interaction of AGEs with cell surface receptors produces superoxide radicals, contributing to oxidative stress and cell damage. As mentioned above,

in colon cancer the receptor for AGE expression is linked with metastatic disease. Several methods exist to dose AGEs, each of which has limitations. In at least one study, HbA_{1c} had the closest relationship with clinical complications of diabetes, when compared with N^ε-carboxymethyllysine and pentosidine, as AGE products were mainly influenced by the quality of diabetes control [52]. The *receptor for advanced glycation end-products (RAGE)* is a member of the immunoglobulin superfamily. It binds multiple ligands, such as AGEs, β-amyloid, and, of interest to cancer progression, amphoterin [53]. This binding triggers a sustained period of cellular activation. The receptor exists at low levels in normal tissues except for lung tissue and becomes upregulated where its ligands accumulate. RAGE is implicated in a broad spectrum of diabetic complications. In the animal, blocking RAGE activation by using soluble RAGE appears to prevent or decrease complications. Colon cancer cells express RAGE, and its ligation activates the ras pathway [54]. RAGE positivity was observed in 19, 81, and 100% of Dukes B, C, and D colorectal cancers in nondiabetic patients [55]. Amphoterin was expressed in most tumors regardless of stage. Animal experiments suggest that RAGE binding to amphoterin in the tumor bed enhances cell migration and invasion, while not markedly altering cell viability and angiogenesis, and that RAGE blockade creates less invasive phenotypes [53]. Binding of AGEs to RAGE appears genotoxic via oxidative mechanisms [56]. Therefore, one can hypothesize that RAGE upregulation and binding could be a potential mechanism by which metabolic syndrome worsens the prognosis of colon cancer, and could be targeted with inhibitors such as sRAGE or RAGE Fab′. RAGE is also overexpressed in other cancers, such as pancreatic and prostate cancers. Notable exceptions are lung and esophageal cancer, in which a higher stage is associated with a downregulation of RAGE.

(4) Animals and humans with metabolic syndrome have a markedly decreased activation of the *atypical PKC-ζ* in their muscle, but not in their liver. PKC-ζ is implicated in glucose uptake, apoptosis, and is also an activator of JUN-B, and therefore is connected to the VEGF signaling pathway. With failure of muscle glucose uptake, resultant hyperinsulinemia increases activity of liver PKC-ζ, which controls lipid synthesis. Thus, lipid production by liver is increased, thereby causing VLDL-associated hypertriglyceridemia and reciprocal decreases in HDL lipids. On the other hand, PKB/Akt activity in the liver is diminished as the metabolic syndrome worsens and this loss of PKB/Akt activation leads to increases in hepatic glucose output, and therefore contributes to hyperglycemia and the appearance of overt diabetes.

The level of PKC-ζ and its responsiveness to insulin, IGF-1 and other growth factors in cancer cells of patients with metabolic syndrome is unknown. Whether insulin/IGF-1 action is impaired or enhanced in cancer cells is uncertain. As antiapoptotic factors that further increase glucose uptake and VEGF production, PKC-ζ and PKB may both be particularly important in tumor progression and metastatic activity. Interestingly, treatment with oral antidiabetics such as rosiglitazone and metformin increases muscle AMPK activity and this restores PKC-ζ activity in skeletal muscle. These muscle insulin sensitizers diminish hyperinsulinemia and this may decrease insulin-dependent actions in cancer cells [57–59]. On the other hand, atypical PKC-ζ might also impair tumorigenesis by repressing IL-6 production [60]. The closely related atypical PKC-ι/λ has also been described as an oncogene, but the impact of metabolic syndrome on its level in humans is unknown [61, 62].

(5) *Leptin and adiponectin.* Obese patients have increased levels of leptin and decreased levels of adiponectin compared to normal weight subjects [47]. Adiponectin is also reduced in diabetic individuals [63]. Leptin mediates the feeling of satiety, improves insulin resistance and hyperglycemia. Obese people appear to demonstrate leptin resistance [64]. Adiponectin regulates energy homeostasis, glucose and lipid metabolism, and has anti-inflammatory and anti-angiogenic properties. Breast cancer patients with metabolic syndrome have higher levels of leptin in their mammary tissue and higher levels of leptin receptors on their tumors than obese patients without metabolic syndrome [65].

(6) *Vascular damage and VEGF.* As noted above, the levels of VEGF may be increased in metabolic syndrome patients [66–68]. VEGF is a key promoter and sustainer of the tumoral neovascularization. Its inhibition by bevacizumab prolongs the survival of metastatic colon cancer patients [69].

(7) *Insulin-mediated vascular proliferation.* Peritumoral vessels overexpress the insulin receptor [48, 70]. In vitro and in vivo experiments demonstrated that insulin can stimulate angiogenesis [70, 71]. These effects occur independently of VEGF/VEGFR signaling, but are dependent upon the insulin receptor itself. Downstream signaling pathways involve PI3K, AKT, sterol regulatory element-binding protein 1 (SREBP-1) and Rac1 [71]. Zhang et al. [72] showed that IR downregulated cancer cells induced xenograft tumors in mice had reduced growth, angiogenesis, lymphangiogensis and metastasis compared with wild-type cells xenografts.

(8) *Inflammation.* Patients with metabolic syndrome are in a state of chronic low-level inflammation. Their IL-6 levels are elevated [73]. Their ability to produce the anti-inflammatory cytokine IL-10 appears impaired [74, 75]. Levels of IL-6 increase with age as well. To what extent this is an effect of age itself, or of the accumulation of clinical and subclinical morbidity is debated [76]. These high levels of IL-6 appear to be associated with insulin resistance and prognosis in colon cancer patients as well [77–79].

(9) *Impaired immunity.* Patients with metabolic syndrome have a decreased cellular immunity [80]. In this study, half of patients had thyroid dysfunction. In patients with normal thyroid function, there was a low relative number of CD3 cells, and hypergammaglobulinemia. There was a close correlation between the levels of free T_3 and CD3, CD4, and CD8 lymphocytes, and an inverse correlation of free T_4 with IgA and IgG levels. It should be noted that intratumoral immune modulation likely plays a large role in immunologic tumoral control. For example, increased amphoterin expression is associated with a depletion of tumor-infiltrating macrophages in colon cancer [81].

(10) *The peroxisome proliferator-activated receptors (PPAR).* The three PPARs (α, β/δ, γ) are nuclear hormone receptors interacting with multiple cellular pathways. PPAR-γ is overexpressed in the muscle of obese and type 2 diabetic subjects and this is insulin-induced [82]. Activation of PPAR-γ by thiazolinediones improves insulin sensitivity, has an antiproliferative effect on cancer cells in vitro, and an anti-inflammatory effect. In a cohort of diabetic veterans, thiazolinediones users had a 33% reduction in risk of lung cancer. In another cohort study, the use of rosiglitazone or pioglitazone by diabetic patients was associated with a decrease in the risk of liver cancer, but not lung and bladder cancer. Rosiglitazone was associated with a decreased risk of colon cancer [83]. The risk of colon and prostate cancer was not statistically different [84]. Chronic activation of PPAR-α can induce hepatocellular carcinoma in rats [85]. PPAR-β/δ is a mediator of EGFR-induced carcinoma cell growth [86]. However, while chemical PPAR agonists have anti-tumoral properties, the link between endogenous overexpression/activation of the receptors and cancer risk in metabolic syndrome patients is unclear at this point.

In summary, metabolic syndrome might favor cancer development and progression via the IGF-1 receptor pathway, hyperinsulinemia itself, hyperglycemia and AGEs, atypical PKC dysregulation, leptin/adiponectin balance alterations, vascular damage and VEGF activation, Insulin-mediated angiogenesis, inflammation, impaired immunity, and/or PPAR modulation. These effects might be compounded in the elderly by synergistic aging-related changes such as higher free IGF-1 and IGF-R levels, increase in AGEs, and IL-6 levels. Such a list of potential factors leads to an important question that lends itself to a bench-to-bedside process that we address next.

From Bench to Bedside

Comparative Studies
Since patients with metabolic syndrome cumulate several risk factors, an important clinical question is: what is the dominant mechanism by which metabolic syndrome interferes with cancer? Identifying such a mechanism is important, since it will be the basis to design effective interventions aiming at the right target for maximum impact. For this we need to move back from laboratory models and return to the patients.

Several results point towards hyperinsulinemia itself being the key driver, although uncertainty remains about the dominant downstream mechanism of action. In a follow-up of the Cremona cohort study, insulin resistance was associated with cancer mortality, independently from diabetes, obesity/visceral obesity, and the metabolic syndrome [28]. In a study by Goodwin et al. [87], insulin-related factors and obesity-related variables had a different impact on the prognosis of breast cancer. Baseline hyperinsulinemia had most correlation with progression-free survival and overall survival during the first 5 years, whereas the effect of BMI and leptin levels had a constant but quadratic association with outcome. C-peptide concentrations, which are a measure of insulin secretion, were found to be a stronger predictor of colorectal cancer risk than was the metabolic syndrome [41]. Postprandial insulin [42] and nonfasting C-peptide [41, 43], a measure of hyperinsulinemia rather than insulin-resistance, are stronger predictors of colon cancer risk than is the fasting insulin concentration [42, 44]. Finally, in one study, chronic insulin therapy was associated with a significantly increased risk of colorectal cancer among patients with type 2 diabetes [45]. Our group conducted a pilot in colorectal cancer patients undergoing their initial surgery. We assessed group differences between metabolic syndrome patients (WHO definition) and those without. We explored six potential mechanisms: hyperinsulinemia, hyperglycemia, increased VEGF levels, AGE levels and RAGE expression, IL-6 levels, and immune tumor infiltration. Blood samples were taken before surgery and 6 months after. Tissue samples were taken from the tumor and normal mucosal tissue. Our results indicated plasma insulin levels as the only significant laboratory difference between groups [48]. Of note was also a diffuse overexpression of IGF-1 R in the tumors, and a high level of expression of the vascular insulin receptors in the peritumoral area of many samples in both groups of patients.

Clinical Trials

In the next step building up from bench to bedside, therapeutic trials are under way based on some of the postulated mechanisms of interaction. Several IGF-1 receptor inhibitors are in clinical trials. They subdivide into anti IGF-1 receptor antibodies, such as figitumumab or cixutumumab, or small molecules with dual IGF-1R and IR inhibitory effect. Figitumumab decreased PSA levels in prostate cancer patients [88], but results in lung [89], head and neck [90], and colon [91] cancer patients have been disappointing. A subset of patients with high IGF-1 levels at baseline might benefit [89]. Cixutumab studies have also been focusing on prostate cancer patients, with results that need further evaluation [92, 93]. A sarcoma study suggests activity in liposarcomas with 1 PR and 21 stable diseases in 37 patients [94]. It had no effect in hepatocellular carcinoma [95]. Small molecule inhibitors are in phase I/II studies. A major side effect of IGF-1 pathway inhibition is the feedback hyperglycemia can potentially cause hyperinsulinemia and dampen the anti-tumor effect of the primary therapy. This might be an issue in metabolic syndrome patients who already have an impaired glucose tolerance [89]. Since hyperinsulinemia by itself might have direct proliferative effects, strategies aiming primarily at a reduction of insulin levels might be of interest. Several studies are testing the impact of metformin. Biguanides prolong survival, delay cancer, and reduce its incidence in animal models [96]. A retrospective study did demonstrate an increased response rate to neoadjuvant chemotherapy in diabetic breast cancer patients receiving metformin [97]. Likewise, retrospective cohorts reveal a 30% improvement in overall survival for colorectal and pancreatic cancer patients with a diabetes treated with metformin [98, 99]. Presently, a large multicentric phase III trial – MA.32 – is testing metformin versus placebo in women receiving adjuvant treatment for their breast cancer. This study does not include diabetic patients, but does stratify patients by body mass index. Thiazolinediones have also been tested for their anti-tumoral properties. A clinical trial randomized 106 men with prostate cancer and rising PSA to rosiglitazone versus placebo [100]. Treated diabetics were excluded. There was no difference in PSA doubling time or time to progression. A small phase II study of rosiglitazone in liposarcoma patients did not find a correlation between PPAR mRNA induction and clinical response [101].

Conclusions

The bedside-to-bench-to-bedside approach illustrated here in the context of metabolic syndrome and cancer can be extended to other comorbidities such as cardiovascular or inflammatory diseases. They illustrate how the coexistence of several diseases in a population of older patients can provide unique insights in the mechanisms of aging and cancer and contribute to the broader field of oncology by uncovering unique unsuspected mechanisms that can be approached with targeted therapies.

References

1. Ford ES, Giles WH, Dietz WH: Prevalence of the metabolic syndrome among US adults: findings from the Third National Health and Nutrition Examination Survey. JAMA 2002;287:356–359.
2. Coughlin SS, Calle EE, Teras LR, et al: Diabetes mellitus as a predictor of cancer mortality in a large cohort of US adults. Am J Epidemiol 2004;159:1160–1167.
3. Hu FB, Manson JE, Liu S, et al: Prospective study of adult onset diabetes mellitus (type 2) and risk of colorectal cancer in women. J Natl Cancer Inst 1999;91:542–547.
4. Meyerhardt JA, Catalano PJ, Haller DG, et al: Impact of diabetes mellitus on outcomes in patients with colon cancer. J Clin Oncol 2003;21:433–440.
5. Varlotto J, Medford-Davis LN, Recht A, et al: Confirmation of the role of diabetes in the local recurrence of surgically resected non-small cell lung cancer. Lung Cancer 2012;75:381–390.
6. Chen CQ, Fang LK, Cai SR, et al: Effects of diabetes mellitus on prognosis of the patients with colorectal cancer undergoing resection: a cohort study with 945 patients. Chin Med J (Engl) 2010;123:3084–3088.
7. Patterson RE, Flatt SW, Saquib N, et al: Medical comorbidities predict mortality in women with a history of early stage breast cancer. Breast Cancer Res Treat 2010;122:859–865.
8. Peairs KS, Barone BB, Snyder CF, et al: Diabetes mellitus and breast cancer outcomes: a systematic review and meta-analysis. J Clin Oncol 2011;29:40–46.
9. Schrauder MG, Fasching PA, Haberle L, et al: Diabetes and prognosis in a breast cancer cohort. J Cancer Res Clin Oncol 2011;137:975–983.
10. Edlinger M, Strohmaier S, Jonsson H, et al: Blood pressure and other metabolic syndrome factors and risk of brain tumour in the large population-based Me-Can cohort study. J Hypertens 2012;30:290–296.
11. Rosato V, Bosetti C, Talamini R, et al: Metabolic syndrome and the risk of breast cancer in postmenopausal women. Ann Oncol 2011;22:2687–2692.
12. Ulmer H, Bjorge T, Concin H, et al: Metabolic risk factors and cervical cancer in the metabolic syndrome and cancer project (Me-Can). Gynecol Oncol 2012;125:330–335.
13. Stocks T, Lukanova A, Bjorge T, et al: Metabolic factors and the risk of colorectal cancer in 580,000 men and women in the metabolic syndrome and cancer project (Me-Can). Cancer 2011;117:2398–2407.
14. Aleksandrova K, Boeing H, Jenab M, et al: Metabolic syndrome and risks of colon and rectal cancer: the European prospective investigation into cancer and nutrition study. Cancer Prev Res (Phila) 2011;4:1873–1883.

15 Kabat GC, Kim MY, Peters U, et al: A longitudinal study of the metabolic syndrome and risk of colorectal cancer in postmenopausal women. Eur J Cancer Prev 2012;21:326–332.

16 Brauer PM, McKeown-Eyssen GE, Jazmaji V, et al: Familial aggregation of diabetes and hypertension in a case-control study of colorectal neoplasia. Am J Epidemiol 2001;156:702–713.

17 Welzel TM, Graubard BI, Zeuzem S, et al: Metabolic syndrome increases the risk of primary liver cancer in the United States: a study in the SEER-Medicare database. Hepatology 2011;54:463–471.

18 Borena W, Strohmaier S, Lukanova A, et al: Metabolic risk factors and primary liver cancer in a prospective study of 578,700 adults. Int J Cancer 2012;131:193–200.

19 Johansen D, Stocks T, Jonsson H, et al: Metabolic factors and the risk of pancreatic cancer: a prospective analysis of almost 580,000 men and women in the Metabolic Syndrome and Cancer Project. Cancer Epidemiol Biomarkers Prev 2010; 19:2307–2317.

20 Rosato V, Tavani A, Bosetti C, et al: Metabolic syndrome and pancreatic cancer risk: a case-control study in Italy and meta-analysis. Metabolism 2011; 60:1372–1378.

21 Pelucchi C, Serraino D, Negri E, et al: The metabolic syndrome and risk of prostate cancer in Italy. Ann Epidemiol 2011;21:835–841.

22 Pasanisi P, Berrino F, De Petris M, et al: Metabolic syndrome as a prognostic factor for breast cancer recurrences. Int J Cancer 2006;119:236–238.

23 Colangelo LA, Gapstur SM, Gann PH, et al: Colorectal cancer mortality and factors related to the insulin resistance syndrome. Cancer Epidemiol Biomarkers Prev 2002;11:385–391.

24 Healy LA, Howard JM, Ryan AM, et al: Metabolic syndrome and leptin are associated with adverse pathological features in male colorectal cancer patients. Colorectal Dis 2012;14:157–165.

25 Flanagan J, Gray PK, Hahn N, et al: Presence of the metabolic syndrome is associated with shorter time to castration-resistant prostate cancer. Ann Oncol 2011;22:801–807.

26 Castillejos-Molina R, Rodriguez-Covarrubias F, Sotomayor M, et al: Impact of metabolic syndrome on biochemical recurrence of prostate cancer after radical prostatectomy. Urol Int 2011;87:270–275.

27 Akbaraly TN, Kivimaki M, Ancelin ML, et al: Metabolic syndrome, its components, and mortality in the elderly. J Clin Endocrinol Metab 2010;95: E327–E332.

28 Perseghin G, Calori G, Lattuada G, et al: Insulin resistance/hyperinsulinemia and cancer mortality: the Cremona study at the 15th year of follow-up. Acta Diabetol 2012, E-pub ahead of print.

29 Hakam A, Yeatman TJ, Lu L, et al: Expression of insulin-like growth factor-1 receptor in human colorectal cancer. Hum Pathol 1999;30:1128–1133.

30 Weber MM, Fottner C, Liu SB, et al: Overexpression of the insulin-like growth factor I receptor in human colon carcinomas. Cancer 2002;95:2086–2095.

31 Sekharam M, Zhao H, Sun M, et al: Insulin-like growth factor-1 receptor enhances invasion and induces resistance to apoptosis of colon cancer cells through the Akt/Bcl-x(L) pathway. Cancer Res 2003;63:7708–7716.

32 Reinmuth N, Liu W, Fan F, et al: Blockade of insulin-like growth factor I receptor function inhibits growth and angiogenesis of colon cancer. Clin Cancer Res 2002;8:3259–3269.

33 Delafontaine P, Song YH, Li Y: Expression, regulation, and function of IGF-1, IGF-1R, and IGF-1 binding proteins in blood vessels. Arterioscler Thromb Vasc Biol 2004;24:435–444.

34 Gapstur SM, Kopp P, Chiu BC, et al: Longitudinal associations of age, anthropometric and lifestyle factors with serum total insulin-like growth factor-I and IGF binding protein-3 levels in Black and White men: the CARDIA Male Hormone Study. Cancer Epidemiol Biomarkers Prev 2004;13: 2208–2216.

35 Janssen JA, Stolk RP, Pols HA, et al: Serum-free IGF-I, total IGF-I, IGFBP-1 and IGFBP-3 levels in an elderly population: relation to age and sex steroid levels. Clin Endocrinol 1998;48:471–478.

36 Raynaud-Simon A: Levels of plasma insulin-like growth factor I (IGF I), IGF II, IGF binding proteins, type 1 IGF receptor and growth hormone binding protein in community-dwelling elderly subjects with no malnutrition and no inflammation. J Nutr Health Aging 2003;7:267–273.

37 Lemne C, Brismar K: Insulin-like growth factor binding protein-1 as a marker of the metabolic syndrome – a study in borderline hypertension. Blood Press 1998;7:89–95.

38 Janssen JA, Lamberts SW: The role of IGF-I in the development of cardiovascular disease in type 2 diabetes mellitus: is prevention possible? Eur J Endocrinol 2002;146:467–477.

39 Sandhu MS, Dunger DB, Giovannucci EL: Insulin, insulin-like growth factor-I (IGF-I), IGF binding proteins, their biologic interactions, and colorectal cancer. J Natl Cancer Inst 2002;94:972–980.

40 Hu FB, Manson JE, Liu S, et al: Prospective study of adult onset diabetes mellitus (type 2) and risk of colorectal cancer in women. J Natl Cancer Inst 1999;91:542–547.

41 Ma J, Pollak MN, Giovannucci E, et al: Prospective study of colorectal cancer risk in men and plasma levels of insulin-like growth factor (IGF)-I and IGF-binding protein-3. J Natl Cancer Inst 1999;91: 620–625.

42 Rechler MM: Growth inhibition by insulin-like growth factor (IGF) binding protein-3 – what's IGF got to do with it? Endocrinology 1997;138: 2645–2647.

43 Dy DY, Whitehead RH, Morris DL: SMS 201.995 inhibits in vitro and in vivo growth of human colon cancer. Cancer Res 1992;52:917–923.

44 Pollak MN, Polychronakos C, Guyda H: Somatostatin analogue SMS 201-995 reduces serum IGF-I levels in patients with neoplasms potentially dependent on IGF-I. Anticancer Res 1989;9:889–891.

45 Yang YX, Hennessy S, Lewis JD: Insulin therapy and colorectal cancer risk among type 2 diabetes mellitus patients. Gastroenterology 2004;127:1044–1050.

46 Lee WM, Lu S, Medline A, et al: Susceptibility of lean and obese Zucker rats to tumorigenesis induced by N-methyl-N-nitrosourea. Cancer Lett 2001; 162:155–160.

47 Braun S, Bitton-Worms K, LeRoith D: The link between the metabolic syndrome and cancer. Int J Biol Sci 2011;7:1003–1015.

48 Liu J, Druta M, Shibata D, et al: Metabolic syndrome and colon cancer: is hyperinsulinemia/insulin receptor-mediated angiogenesis a critical process? J Geriatr Oncol 2011;2:S61.

49 Komninou D, Ayonote A, Richie JP Jr, et al: Insulin resistance and its contribution to colon carcinogenesis. Exp Biol Med (Maywood) 2003;228:396–405.

50 Popovich IG, Zabezhinski MA, Egormin PA, et al: Insulin in aging and cancer: antidiabetic drug Diabenol as geroprotector and anticarcinogen. Int J Biochem Cell Biol 2005;37:1117–1129.

51 Wautier JL, Schmidt AM: Protein glycation: a firm link to endothelial cell dysfunction. Circ Res 2004; 95:233–238.

52 Schiel R, Franke S, Appel T, et al: Improvement in quality of diabetes control and concentrations of AGE products in patients with type 1 and insulin-treated type 2 diabetes mellitus studied over a period of 10 years (JEVIN). J Diabetes Complications 2003;17:90–97.

53 Schmidt AM, Yan SD, Yan SF, et al: The multiligand receptor RAGE as a progression factor amplifying immune and inflammatory responses. J Clin Invest 2001;108:949–955.

54 Zill H, Gunther R, Erbersdobler HF, et al: RAGE expression and AGE-induced MAP kinase activation in Caco-2 cells. Biochem Biophys Res Commun 2001;288:1108–1111.

55 Kuniyasu H, Chihara Y, Takahashi T: Co-expression of receptor for advanced glycation end products and the ligand amphoterin associates closely with metastasis of colorectal cancer. Oncol Rep 2003;10: 445–448.

56 Stopper H, Schinzel R, Sebekova K, et al: Genotoxicity of advanced glycation end products in mammalian cells. Cancer Lett 190:151–156.

57 Beeson M, Sajan MP, Daspet JG, et al: Defective activation of protein kinase C-ζ in muscle by insulin and phosphatidylinositol-3,4,5,-$(PO_4)_3$ in obesity and polycystic ovary syndrome. Metab Syndr Relat Disord 2004;2:49–56.

58 Beeson M, Sajan MP, Dizon M, et al: Activation of protein kinase C-ζ by insulin and phosphatidylinositol-3,4,5-$(PO_4)_3$ is defective in muscle in type 2 diabetes and impaired glucose tolerance: amelioration by rosiglitazone and exercise. Diabetes 2003; 52:1926–1934.

59 Farese RV, Sajan MP, Standaert ML: Atypical protein kinase C in insulin action and insulin resistance. Biochem Soc Trans 2005;33:350–353.

60 Galvez AS, Duran A, Linares JF, et al: Protein kinase C-ζ represses the interleukin-6 promoter and impairs tumorigenesis in vivo. Mol Cell Biol 2009; 29:104–115.

61 Fields AP, Regala RP: Protein kinase C-ι: human oncogene, prognostic marker and therapeutic target. Pharmacol Res 2007;55:487–497.

62 Farese RV, Sajan MP: Metabolic functions of atypical protein kinase C: 'good' and 'bad' as defined by nutritional status. Am J Physiol Endocrinol Metab 2010;298:E385–E394.

63 Berg AH, Combs TP, Scherer PE: ACRP30/adiponectin: an adipokine regulating glucose and lipid metabolism. Trends Endocrinol Metab 2002;13: 84–89.

64 Maffei M, Fei H, Lee GH, et al: Increased expression in adipocytes of ob RNA in mice with lesions of the hypothalamus and with mutations at the db locus. Proc Natl Acad Sci USA 1995;92:6957–6960.

65 Carroll PA, Healy L, Lysaght J, et al: Influence of the metabolic syndrome on leptin and leptin receptor in breast cancer. Mol Carcinog 2011;50: 643–651.

66 Cukiernik M, Hileeto D, Evans T, et al: Vascular endothelial growth factor in diabetes induced early retinal abnormalities. Diabetes Res Clin Pract 2004;65:197–208.

67 Rizkalla B, Forbes JM, Cao Z, et al: Temporal renal expression of angiogenic growth factors and their receptors in experimental diabetes: role of the renin-angiotensin system. J Hypertens 2005;23:153–164.
68 Lim HS, Blann AD, Chong AY, et al: Plasma vascular endothelial growth factor, angiopoietin-1, and angiopoietin-2 in diabetes: implications for cardiovascular risk and effects of multifactorial intervention. Diabetes Care 2004;27:2918–2924.
69 Hurwitz H, Fehrenbacher L, Novotny W, et al: Bevacizumab plus irinotecan, fluorouracil, and leucovorin for metastatic colorectal cancer. N Engl J Med 2004;350:2335–2342.
70 Rensing KL, Houttuijn Bloemendaal FM, Weijers EM, et al: Could recombinant insulin compounds contribute to adenocarcinoma progression by stimulating local angiogenesis? Diabetologia 2010;53:966–970.
71 Liu Y, Petreaca M, Martins-Green M: Cell and molecular mechanisms of insulin-induced angiogenesis. J Cell Mol Med 2009;13:4492–4504.
72 Zhang H, Fagan DH, Zeng X, et al: Inhibition of cancer cell proliferation and metastasis by insulin receptor downregulation. Oncogene 2010;29:2517–2527.
73 Esposito K, Giugliano D: The metabolic syndrome and inflammation: association or causation? Nutr Metab Cardiovasc Dis 2004;14:228–232.
74 Esposito K, Pontillo A, Giugliano F, et al: Association of low interleukin-10 levels with the metabolic syndrome in obese women. J Clin Endocrinol Metab 2003;88:1055–1058.
75 Van Exel E, Gussekloo J, de Craen AJ, et al: Low production capacity of interleukin-10 associates with the metabolic syndrome and type 2 diabetes: The Leiden 85-Plus Study. Diabetes 2002;51:1088–1092.
76 Ferrucci L, Corsi A, Lauretani F, et al: The origins of age-related proinflammatory state. Blood 2005;105:2294–2299.
77 Makino T, Noguchi Y, Yoshikawa T, et al: Circulating interleukin-6 concentrations and insulin resistance in patients with cancer. Br J Surg 1998;85:1658–1662.
78 Belluco C, Nitti D, Frantz M, et al: Interleukin-6 blood level is associated with circulating carcinoembryonic antigen and prognosis in patients with colorectal cancer. Ann Surg Oncol 2000;7:133–138.
79 Galizia G, Orditura M, Romano C, et al: Prognostic significance of circulating IL-10 and IL-6 serum levels in colon cancer patients undergoing surgery. Clin Immunol 2002;102:169–178.
80 Zabelina VD, Zemskov VM, Mkrtumian AM, et al: Characteristics of immune system in patients with metabolic syndrome (in Russian). Ter Arkh 2004;76:66–72.
81 Kuniyasu H, Sasaki T, Sasahira T, et al: Depletion of tumor-infiltrating macrophages is associated with amphoterin expression in colon cancer. J Immunopathol Mol Cell Biol 2004;71:129–136.
82 Park KS, Ciaraldi TP, Abrams-Carter L, et al: PPAR-γ gene expression is elevated in skeletal muscle of obese and type 2 diabetic subjects. Diabetes 1997;46:1230–1234.
83 Chang CH, Lin JW, Wu LC, et al: Association of thiazolidinediones with liver cancer and colorectal cancer in type 2 diabetes mellitus. Hepatology 2012;55:1462–1472.
84 Govindarajan R, Ratnasinghe L, Simmons DL, et al: Thiazolidinediones and the risk of lung, prostate, and colon cancer in patients with diabetes. J Clin Oncol 2007;25:1476–1481.
85 Pyper SR, Viswakarma N, Yu S, et al: PPAR-α: energy combustion, hypolipidemia, inflammation and cancer. Nucl Recept Signal 2010;8:e002.
86 Kannan-Thulasiraman P, Seachrist DD, Mahabeleshwar GH, et al: Fatty acid-binding protein 5 and PPAR-β/δ are critical mediators of epidermal growth factor receptor-induced carcinoma cell growth. J Biol Chem 2010;285:19106–19115.
87 Goodwin PJ, Ennis M, Pritchard KI, et al: Insulin- and obesity-related variables in early-stage breast cancer: correlations and time course of prognostic associations. J Clin Oncol 2012;30:164–171.
88 Chi K, Gleave ME, Fazli L, Goldenberg SL, So A, Kollmannsberger CK, Murray N, Tinker A, Gualberto A, Pollak MN: A phase II study of preoperative figitumumab in patients with localized prostate cancer. J Clin Oncol 2010;28:abstr 4662.
89 Jassem J, Langer CJ, Karp DD, et al: Randomized, open label, phase III trial of figitumumab in combination with paclitaxel and carboplatin versus paclitaxel and carboplatin in patients with non-small cell lung cancer. J Clin Oncol 2010;28:abstr 7500.
90 Schmitz S, Kaminsky-Forrett M, Henry S, et al: Phase II study of figitumumab in patients with recurrent and/or metastatic squamous cell carcinoma of the head and neck: GORTEC 2008–2002. J Clin Oncol 2010;28:abstr 5500.
91 Becerra C, Salazar R, Garcia-Carbonero R, et al: Phase II trial of figitumumab in patients with refractory, metastatic colorectal cancer. J Clin Oncol 2011;29: abstr 3525.

92 Higano C, Alumkal JJ, Ryan CJ, et al: A phase II study of cixutumumab (IMC-A12), a monoclonal antibody against the insulin-like growth factor 1 receptor, monotherapy in metastatic castration-resistant prostate cancer: feasibility of every 3-week dosing and updated results. ASCO Genitourinary Cancers Symposium, 2010:abstr 189.

93 Hussain M, Rathkopf DE, Liu G, et al: A phase II randomized study of cixutumumab (IMC-A12: CIX) or ramucirumab (IMC-1121B: RAM) plus mitoxantrone and prednisone in patients with metastatic castrate-resistant prostate cancer following disease progression on docetaxel therapy. J Clin Oncol 2012;30:abstr 97.

94 Schoffski P AD, Blay J, Gil T, et al: Phase II trial of anti-IGF-IR antibody cixutumumab in patients with advanced or metastatic soft-tissue sarcoma and Ewing family of tumors. J Clin Oncol 2011;29: abstr 10004.

95 Abou-Alfa G, Gansukh B, Chou JF, et al: Phase II study of cixutumumab (IMC-A12, NSC742460;C) in hepatocellular carcinoma. J Clin Oncol 2011;29: abstr 4043.

96 Anisimov VN: The relationship between aging and carcinogenesis: a critical appraisal. Crit Rev Oncol Hematol 2003;45:277–304.

97 Jiralerspong S, Palla SL, Giordano SH, et al: Metformin and pathologic complete responses to neoadjuvant chemotherapy in diabetic patients with breast cancer. J Clin Oncol 2009;27:3297–3302.

98 Sadeghi N, Abbruzzese JL, Yeung SJ, Hassan M, Li D: Effect of metformin on survival of diabetic patients with pancreatic adenocarcinoma. J Clin Oncol 2011;29:abstr 4063.

99 Hassabo H, Hassan M, George B, Wen S, Baladandayuthapani V, Kopetz S, Fogelman DR, Kee BK, Eng C, Garrett CR: Survival advantage associated with metformin usage in patients with colorectal cancer and type 2 noninsulin-dependent diabetes. J Clin Oncol 2011;29:abstr 3618.

100 Smith MR, Manola J, Kaufman DS, et al: Rosiglitazone versus placebo for men with prostate carcinoma and a rising serum prostate-specific antigen level after radical prostatectomy and/or radiation therapy. Cancer 2004;101:1569–1574.

101 Debrock G, Vanhentenrijk V, Sciot R, et al: A phase II trial with rosiglitazone in liposarcoma patients. Br J Cancer 2003;89:1409–1412.

Martine Extermann, MD
Senior Adult Oncology Program
H. Lee Moffitt Cancer Center and Research Institute
University of South Florida
12902 Magnolia Drive, SA-Prog, Tampa, FL 33612 (USA)
E-Mail martine.extermann@moffitt.org

Frailty: A Common Pathway in Aging and Cancer

Lodovico Balducci

Senior Adult Oncology Program, H. Lee Moffitt Cancer Center and Research Institute, University of South Florida, Tampa, Fla., USA

Abstract

The construct of frailty is germane to that of aging, but a clinical definition of frailty is still wanted. In the geriatric literature, frailty has been conceived in two different ways. The first one is a threshold beyond which the functional reserve of a person is critically reduced and the tolerance of stress negligible. The second is as a progressive reduction of functional reserve due to a progressive accumulation of deficit. In this construct it may be hard to distinguish frailty from aging. Neither concept has at present a clear application in the management of older cancer patients. Studies are needed to establish whether the construct of frailty proposed by Fried et al. may be predictive of decreased cancer-independent survival and of decreased treatment tolerance in older cancer patients.

Copyright © 2013 S. Karger AG, Basel

Aging, Cancer, and Frailty

Age and frailty have been associated for a long time in the medical as well as in the lay literature [1]. The idea of frailty conjures images of increased susceptibility to stress, which is also the hallmark of aging, yet it is becoming clearer and clearer that many, may be the majority, of older individuals are able to tolerate a significant amount of stresses without compromise of their life expectancy or of their function [2]. This observation is particularly relevant to cancer treatment. Properly selected older individuals may undergo aggressive treatment without long-lasting consequences. Hence the need to define frailty in more restrictive terms than simple age [3].

There is universal agreement on three areas concerning frailty: (1) Frailty is a condition of critically reduced functional reserve that leads to enhanced vulnerability to stress [1, 4–8]. (2) Frailty is a clinical syndrome that may result from different and interactive mechanisms related to age, including chronic inflammation, sarcopenia, comorbidity, and dysregulation of multiple physiologic systems. The causes of frailty are both environmental and inherited. (3) Frailty is a chronic condition.

Currently, two different constructs of frailty are entertained [1]. According to one, frailty is a phenotype that identifies among functionally independent individuals those at increased risk of death and dependence [5]. Though able of independent living, the frail person may experience both loss of independence and shortening of life expectancy when subjected to a stress that would be negligible for other persons. Examples of these stresses may include elective cancer surgery or standard radiation therapy and chemotherapy. The alternative construct sees frailty as an ongoing decline of one's functional reserve between fully independent living and death. In lieu of a frailty phenotype, this construct identifies different degrees of frailty, assessed as a frailty index [9]. These views are not mutually exclusive but rather represent different ways to recognize and assess frailty. Both of them are tested in the clinical arena to establish whether there are circumstances in which one form of assessment is more appropriate.

In this chapter we will explore the current clinical definitions of frailty and their applications to the management of cancer.

Clinical Definition of Frailty

Physiologic and Chronologic Age
It is commonly accepted that chronologic age is a poor reflection of physiologic age at least up to age 90–95. Physiologic age is defined currently as risk of mortality, and of functional dependence (need of assistance in the activities of daily living) [2]. Frailty may be considered as an intermediate status between independence and functional dependence (fig. 1). In this construct, individuals with functional dependence are in a condition beyond frailty. Alternatively, frailty may be defined as the degree of susceptibility to stress. In this construct even individuals who are already functionally dependent may experience different degrees of frailty, expressed as increasing risk of death and of further functional decline.

Several indices have been developed to estimate one's risk of death and of functional decline that is to assess a person's physiologic age (table 1).

Aging may be seen as a chronic and progressive inflammation [10]. The concentration of inflammatory markers in the circulation may then reflect functional age [11]. In addition to inflammatory cytokines, these markers include products of fibrinolysis and in particular D-dimer, as inflammation is associated with chronic disseminated intravascular coagulation [12, 13]. Interleukin-6 (IL-6) has been the most extensively studied inflammatory cytokine. Its circulatory levels are increased in the presence of virtually all geriatric syndromes, such as dementia, delirium, depression, osteoporosis, and failure to thrive [13]. Almost 10 years ago, Cohen et al. [11] assessed the concentration of D-dimer and IL-6 in individuals who were independent, without significant comorbidity, and lived at home. When the levels of both markers were normal, the risk of functional dependence or death at 10 years was less than 10%.

Fig. 1. Conceptualization of frailty as a phenotype. A mild stress does not affect the function of a fit person, but precipitates functional dependence in a frail one.

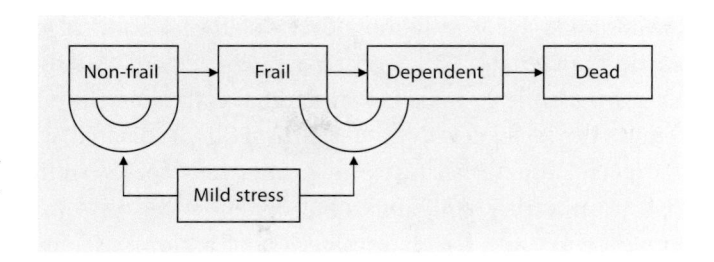

Table 1. Instruments of current use for the assessment of physiologic age

Comprehensive Geriatric Assessment (CGA)
Function expressed as activities of daily living (ADL) and instrumental activities of daily living (IADL)
Comorbidity
Geriatric syndromes
Nutrition
Living conditions and social support
Laboratory tests
    Circulating inflammatory markers
    Length of leukocyte telomeres
Functional examinations
    Timed up-and-go test
Combination
    Allostatic load
    Frailty Index

This risk increased to 20 and 40% respectively when the concentration of one or both substances was increased. The same data demonstrate however that a one-time determination does not have adequate sensitivity to assess the physiologic age of a person, as more than 60% of those with both abnormal markers were alive and independent at 2 years. Furthermore, these markers may not be utilized in the course of acute diseases, as their concentration is likely to be increased in patients of any age. For the same reason, they are of limited utility in patients with advanced cancer that is associated both with inflammation and disseminated intravascular coagulation. It is reasonable to assume that serial levels of these substances may reflect physiologic age as well as rate of aging, in individuals who are otherwise healthy, but this hypothesis has not been confirmed as yet in a clinical investigation.

The length of the leukocyte telomeres also reflects the functional age of a person. Several studies have shown that the shorter the telomeres in patients of the same chronologic age, the higher the risk of death and of other manifestations of aging such as cancer [14, 15], geriatric syndromes [16], and functional dependence [16, 17]. It is impossible to make an individual estimate of functional age based on telomere length, however, due to high interindividual variability.

Several functional tests, including the popular timed 'get up and go' predict the risk of mortality and functional dependence [18]. Most investigators are reluctant however to trust the determination of a complex phenomenon such as aging to a single test. Yet these tests are helpful to predict individual risk of disability. They have not been studied to predict the response to stress including surgery or antineoplastic chemotherapy.

The allostatic load is based on the assumption that age represents a loss of homeostatic control that is of the ability of an organism to reverse to basic levels of function after a stress [19]. It requires the assessment of physical, laboratory, and functional parameters. Chronic inflammation is a form of allostasis and the determination of inflammatory markers in the circulation is indeed an assessment of the allostatic load. This instrument appears too complex for routine clinical use at present.

The frailty index and its many variations are based on the number or the degrees of functional deficits accumulated by a person. In its original form the frailty index may provide the most accurate determination of physiologic age (fig. 2) [20]. It appears too laborious for clinical use though, as it involves the assessment of about 70 parameters including disease, loss of physical function and of social support.

The Comprehensive Geriatric Assessment (CGA) including function, expressed as instrumental activities of daily living (IADL) and activities of daily living (ADL), comorbidity, presence or absence of geriatric syndromes, represents the best validated instrument for the determination of mortality risk [2, 21] and of stress tolerance [22–24]. Figure 3 illustrates how these elements can be integrated in a prediction of mortality risk for people aged 50–90 [21]. Elements of the CGA, and in particular dependence in one or more IADL, are also predictive of the complication of cancer surgery and cancer chemotherapy [22–25].

Frailty and Aging. Frailty Phenotype
If frailty is considered an intermediate status between independent aging and functional dependence, it should be possible to identify a frailty phenotype [5] or a frailty syndrome [8] using the same parameters that reflect physiologic aging.

The frailty phenotype first described by Fried et al. [5] is still considered by many as the golden standard of frailty (table 2). It was obtained from an analysis of the data of the Cardiovascular Health Study (CHS), a longitudinal study of more than 8,500 individuals aged 65 and over for an average of 11 years. The individuals belonging to the three-phenotype non-frail, pre-frail, and frail had a different risk of mortality, of functional dependence, of hospitalization and of admission to assisted living over a median 8-year follow-up. In the Woman Health and Aging Study II involving 707 women aged 70–79, Fried et al. [5] analyzed the relation between the frailty phenotype

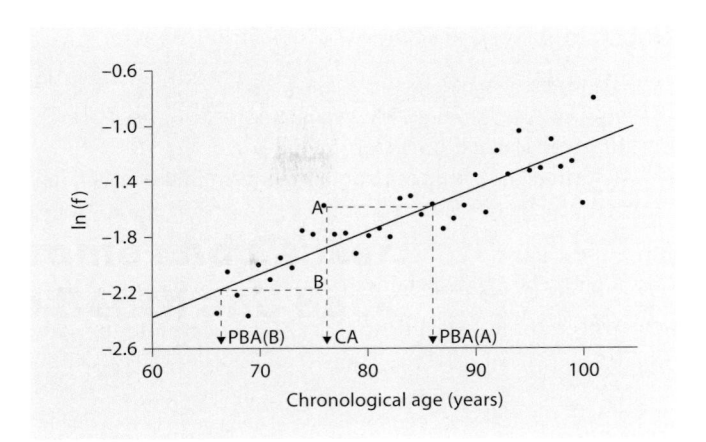

Fig. 2. Determination of an individual's physiologic age based on frailty index. From Mitnitski et al. [20], with permission.

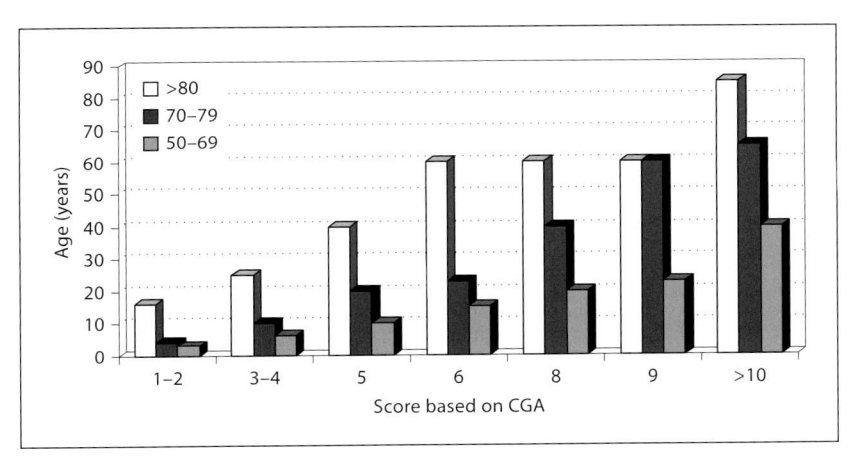

Fig. 3. Four-year mortality estimate of patients in different age groups according to a score based on CGA [21].

and allostasis [26]. They found that individuals judged frail and pre-frail had a four- and twofold increased risk respectively to have three or more comorbid conditions or dysregulation of three or more physiologic systems with respect to those who were fit. Thus the phenotype may be considered a reflection of both comorbidity and physiologic abnormalities. More recently the authors established a relationship between frailty and comorbidity in the CHS [27]. They found that frailty was associated with depression, stroke, dementia, arthritis, and pulmonary diseases, and disease burden attenuated the association between frailty and age. In other words, disease burden was an independent risk factor for frailty.

Table 2. Elements that define the CHS frailty phenotype

- Involuntary weight loss ≥10 lb in 6 months
- Decreased grip strength for sex and age
- Decreased walking speed for sex and age
- Exhaustion, measured as two statements from the CES-D depression scale
- Physical activity, measured on the short version of the Minnesota Leisure Time activity (see below): men <383 kcal/week, females <270 kcal/week

Grip strength by BMI (BMI derived from height and body surface)

BMI	cut-off grip strength (kg)
Male	
<24	<29
24.1–26	<30
26.1–28	<30
28	<32
Female	
<23	<17
23.1–26	<17.3
26.1–29	<18
>29	<21

Walk time

Height	cut-off point (s)
Men	
<173 cm	>7
>173 cm	>6
Women	
<159 cm	>7
>159 cm	>6

Exhaustion: score 2 or 3 on two questions of the CES-D
    a. I felt everything I did was an effort
    b. I could not get going
Scores: 0 = never; 1 = 1–2 days/week; 2 = 3–4 days/week; 3 = most of the time

Physical activity: Patients will be asked whether they engaged in any of the following activity in the past 2 weeks:

High-intensity activities	*Moderate or light-intensity activity*
Swimming	Gardening, mowing, raking
Hiking	Golfing
Anaerobics	Bowling
Tennis	Biking
Jogging	Dancing
Racquetball	Calisthenics
Walked for exercise for at least 1 h >4 mph	Exercise cycle
	Walked for exercise for at least 1 h at a strolling pace

Patients who did not engage in any of these activities over the past 2 weeks will be considered at low physical activity

Table 2. continued

Non-frail: no abnormality present
Pre-frail: 1–2 abnormalities
Frail: ≥3 abnormalities

A number of modifications of the original phenotype have been proposed including the insertion of IL-6 levels [28] and of cognitive decline [29] among the assessment parameters. It is not clear at present if they present any advantage with respect to the original phenotype.

The importance of the CHS definition cannot be overstated as it was the first successful attempt to predict different outcomes in functional aging individuals. It definitely identifies individuals with different functional reserve based on a simple phenotype. It also provides a reference to study the possibility to reverse or delay the aging process by focusing the effort on individuals who are pre-frail and frail.

It is legitimate to ask whether these criteria really define frailty and how much they need to be fine tuned. After a follow-up of 8 years, 60% of the so-called 'frail' and 75% of the so-called pre-frail individuals were still alive, and a significant portion of them were still living independently. So far there is no direct evidence that frail or pre-frail individuals are more susceptible to stress than the non-frail ones. Kristjansson et al. [24] studied the predictive value for surgical complications and survival in 172 cancer patients aged 70–94. The phenotype predicted survival but not the risk of surgical complications that were best predicted by dependence in ADL or presence of a geriatric syndrome. The frailty phenotype does not seem to be as sensitive as the CGA in estimating the risk of therapeutic complications, at least in surgical patients.

More recently an alternative frailty phenotype has been proposed by the investigators of the osteoporosis by the investigators of the Study of Osteoporotic Fractures (SOF) in older men [30, 31]. This phenotype that has been inappropriately called index, is based on three elements: weight loss, inability to raise from a chair five times without using the arms, and exhaustion. Individuals are classified as robust (no abnormalities), intermediates (1 abnormality) and frail (2 or more abnormalities). In 3,132 men aged 67 and over [30] and in 735 men and women aged 70–79 [31], the predictive accuracy of the CHS and the SOF phenotype were compared. A ROC showed that both phenotypes were equally reliable in predicting death, disability, hospitalization, and institutionalization. The SOF instrument is very appealing as it is much simpler to assess than the CHS one. However, the SOF follow-up is only 3 years.

Frailty Indices

A group of Canadian investigators proposed an index based on 70 'deficits in health' obtained from the assessment of 10,263 individuals included in the first Canadian Study of Health and Aging (CSHA1) [32]. Deficits included diseases, dependence in ADL and IADL, physical and neurological signs and symptoms, laboratory tests and radiographic examinations. The index was obtained by dividing by 100 the number of deficits. For example, if a person had 7 deficits, his/her frailty index would have been 0.07. This index proved to be very accurate in predicting the individual risk of death and institutionalization. Comparing the index in individual subjects with the average index of subjects of the same chronologic age, that authors devised for the first time an assessment of the so-called 'physiologic age' [20]. The authors and others also demonstrated that frailty indices obtained from patients' self-reports were equally reliable [21, 33–36] even when different deficits from those originally described were included and even when it was based on subjects' self-reports. Recently the same investigators established some standard procedures for creating a frailty index [37–39]. In a secondary analysis of the Yale Precipitating Event Project (PEP) in which 754 elderly aged 70 and over were included, they established five criteria to select a deficit as well as a grading of the severity of each deficit. In 2 cohorts of patient the indices proved highly reproducible as well as highly predictive of mortality and survival. The authors emphasized that the frailty index is not meant as a model to predict the risk of mortality, but as an instrument to describe the degree of vulnerability of older individuals to stress. This intention is reflected in the five criteria to select the parameters that compose the index. In particular, the items selected need to cover a wide range of systems. For example, not more than two or three deficits should be pertaining at the same domain (cognition, motility, muscular strength, etc.), whereas in a pure mortality index all the items that predict mortality independently should be included.

In an analysis of a subgroup of 4,721 individuals included in the CHS, the investigators of Duke University demonstrated that a frailty index based on 48 deficits was more accurate in predicting the mortality risk than the frailty phenotype [40]. In particular, among the 1,073 frail individuals, according to the phenotypic classification, the phenotypic classification underestimated the risk of death for 720 and the frailty index for 134.

Aware of the fact that a frailty index may be too laborious for a busy clinical practice and may also be redundant, the Canadian investigators have also proposed the use of frailty scales. The first of these scales scored elderly individuals from 0 through 3. Those scored as 0 had the lowest and those scored 3 the highest risk of mortality and functional dependence over 80 months' follow-up. The scale was obtained from a retrospective analysis of a random sample of 9,008 community residents aged 65+ included in the Canadian provincial comprehensive sampling frame. It was based on presence of incontinence, dementia, dependence in IADL and ADL [41]. More recently, they proposed a scale of frailty based on pure clinical impression (table 3) [42]: 30 family physicians, 30 geriatricians and internists, 11

Table 3. Scale of fitness and frailty based on clinical impression

1.	Very fit
2.	Well – person without active disease but who does not appear as active and energetic as the fit one
3.	Well – with treated comorbid diseases
4.	Apparently vulnerable – independent but complaining of fatigue and of symptoms related to disease
5.	Mildly frail – dependent in some IADL
6.	Moderately frail – dependent in both ADL and IADL
7.	Frail – completely dependent on others or terminally ill

neurologists and 6 psychiatrists were asked to do a clinical evaluation of a subgroup of 2,305 subjects of the CAHS and to classify them according to the scale. The clinical impression was highly predictive of mortality and functional dependence and bore a close relationship with the original frailty index.

Frailty and Vulnerability

The term 'vulnerability' has been frequently used in the geriatric literature [43]. The relationship between frailty and vulnerability is not clear. The term has been used in two contexts. The first is to describe a condition of aging associated with increased risk of mortality and functional dependence that is identified and scored with the Vulnerable Elders Survey-13 (VES-13). This survey includes 13 items, given a different weight, and the final score predicts the risk of adverse outcome. In this respect, vulnerability is conceptually identical to frailty and the VES-13 may be considered as a form of frailty index.

The second context includes a number of health domains, such as falls, incontinence, impair mobility or cognitive decline where age is a risk factor for impairment [44] and that should represent a special focus of care for older individuals [45]. In this construct, vulnerability is an attribute of aging that should be used to direct the care as well as to assess the quality of care of older individuals [46]. In this context, vulnerability is clearly distinct for frailty as it is defined as an area of intervention rather than as a clinical syndrome.

Frailty and Cancer

Cancer is a disease of aging and frailty is an aging-related syndrome. The interactions of cancer and frailty are then of interest to the practitioner. In particular one may ask:

(1) Is cancer a cause of frailty? (2) Is cancer treatment a cause of frailty? (3) Is frailty a risk factor for the complications of cancer treatment? (4) Is frailty reversible with the treatment of cancer?

While it is reasonable to assume that cancer and cancer treatment may cause frailty and that frail individuals are more susceptible to the complications of both cancer and cancer treatment, these hypotheses were never proved. In part, the confusion related to the definition and the assessment of frailty may be responsible for the scarcity of data related to aging and cancer.

In the meantime one may ask how the definition of a frailty phenotype (or of a frailty syndrome) and how the determination of a frailty index may impact the treatment of cancer in the older aged person. Recent studies have shown that the CGA may be utilized to predict the risk of mortality [2, 21], and the risk of surgical and chemotherapy complications [22–25]. Seemingly, the CGA may be utilized as well to monitor the medical, functional, emotional and cognitive consequences of cancer and cancer treatment. Only future clinical studies will tell us whether the determination of frailty may add unique information to that already provided by current instruments. Certainly the assessment of the risk of mortality and therapeutic complications needs to be made both simpler and more accurate, but it is not clear whether the assessment of frailty is the proper instrument toward this goal.

References

1 Lacas A, Rockwood K: Frailty in primary care: a review of its conceptualizations and implications for practice. BMC Med 2012;10:4–27.
2 Yourman LC, Lee SJ, Schonberg MA, et al: Prognostic indices for older adults: a systematic review. JAMA 2012;307:182–192.
3 Mariano J, Min LC: Assessment; in Naeim A, Reuben DB, Ganz PA (eds): Management of Cancer in the Older Patient. Philadelphia, Elsevier Saunders, 2012, pp 39–50.
4 Sternberg SA, Wershof-Schwarz A, Karunananthan S, et al: The identification of frailty: a systematic literature review. J Am Geriatr Soc 2011;59:2129–2138.
5 Fried LP, Tangen CM, Walston J, et al: Frailty in older adults: evidence of a phenotype. J Gerontol A Biol Sci Med Sci 2001;56:146–156.
6 Quinlan N, Marcantonio NR, Inoyou SK, et al: Vulnerability: the crossroads of frailty and delirium. J Am Geriatr Soc 2011;59(suppl 2):S262–S268.
7 Mohile SG, Xian W, Dale W, et al: Association of a cancer diagnosis with vulnerability and frailty in older Medicare beneficiaries. J Natl Cancer Inst 2009;101:1206–1215.
8 Xue QL: The frailty syndrome, definition and natural history. Clin Geriatr Med 2011;27:1–15.
9 Rockwood K, Mitnitski A: Frailty, fitness and the mathematics of deficit accumulation. Rev Clin Gerontol 2007;17:1–12.
10 Ferrucci L, Corsi A, Lauretani F, et al: The origin of age-related pro-inflammatory state. Blood 2005; 105:2294–2299.
11 Cohen HJ, Harris T, Pieper CF: Coagulation and activation of inflammatory pathways in the development of functional decline and mortality in the elderly. Am J Med 2003;114:180–187.
12 McBane RD, Hardison AM, Sobel BE, et al: Comparison of levels of plasminogen activator inhibitor-1, tissue type plasminogen activator antigen, fibrinogen and D-dimer in various age decades in patients with type 2 diabetes mellitus and stable coronary artery disease. Am J Cardiol 2010;105:17–24.
13 Kanapuru B, Ershler WB: Inflammation, coagulation, and the pathway to frailty. Am J Med 2009; 122:605–613.

14 Willeit P, Willeit J, Kloss-Blandstätter A, et al: Fifteen-year follow-up of the association between telomere length and incident cancer and cancer mortality. JAMA 2011;306:42–44.
15 Ma H, Zou Z, Wei S, et al: Shortened telomere length is associated with increased risk of cancer: a meta-analysis. PLoS One 2011;6:e20466.
16 Zhu H, Belcher M, Van der Harst P: Healthy aging and disease: role for telomere biology. Clin Sci (Lond) 2011;120:427–440.
17 Mather KA, Jorm AF, Parslow RA, et al: Is telomere length a biomarker of aging? A review. J Gerontol A Biol Sci Med Sci 2011;66:202–213.
18 Botolfsen P, Helbostad JL, Moe-Nillsen R, et al: Reliability and concurrent validity of the expanded timed up-and-go test in older people with impaired mobility. Physiother Res Int 2008;13:94–106.
19 Grunewald TM, Seeman TE, Karlamangla AS, et al: Allostatic load and frailty in older adults. J Am Geriatr Soc 2009;57:1525–1531.
20 Mitniski AB, Song X, Rockwood K: The assessment of relative fitness or frailty in community-dwelling older adults using self-report data. J Gerontol A Biol Sci Med Sci 2004;59:M627–M632.
21 Lee SJ, Lindquist K, Segal MR, et al: Development and validation of a prognostic index for 4-year mortality in older adults. JAMA 2006;295:801–808.
22 Hurria A, Togawa K, Mohile SG, et al: Predicting chemotherapy toxicity in older adults with cancer. J Clin Oncol 2011;29:3457–3465.
23 Extermann M, Boler I, Reich RR, et al: Predicting the risk of chemotherapy toxicity in older patients: The Chemotherapy Toxicity Assessment Scale in High Age Patients (CRASH) score. Cancer 2012;118:3377–3386.
24 Kristjansson SR, Rønning B, Hurria A, et al: A comparison of two preoperative frailty measures in older surgical cancer patients. J Geriatr Oncol 2012;3:1–7.
25 Kristjansson SR, Nesbakken A, Jordy MS, et al: Comprehensive Geriatric Assessment can predict complications in elderly patients after elective surgery for colorectal cancer: a prospective observation cohort study. Crit Rev Oncol Hematol 2010;76:208–217.
26 Fried LP, Xiu QL, Cappola AR, et al: Nonlinear multisystem physiological dysregulation associated with frailty in older women. Implications for etiology and treatment. J Gerontol A Biol Sci Med Sci 2009;64:1049–1057.
27 Sanders JL, Boudreau RM, Fried LP, et al: Measurement of organ structure and function enhances understanding of the physiological basis of frailty: the Cardiovascular Health Study. J Am Geriatr Soc 2012;59:1581–1588.
28 Sarkisian CA, Gruenewald TL, John Boscardin W, et al: Preliminary evidence for sub-dimensions of geriatric frailty: the MacArthur study of successful aging. J Am Geriatr Soc 2008;56:2292–2297.
29 Avila-Funes JA, Amieva A, Barbager-Gateau P, et al: Cognitive impairment improves the predictive ability of frailty for adverse health outcomes: the three city study. J Am Geriatr Soc 2009;57:453–461.
30 Ensrud KE, Ewing SK, Cawthon PM, et al: A comparison of frailty indices for the prediction of falls disability, fractures and mortality in older men. J Am Geriatr Soc 2009;57:492–498.
31 Kiely DK, Cupples LA, Lipsitz LA: Validation and comparison of two frailty indexes: the MOBILIZE Boston Study. J Am Geriatr Soc 2009;57:1032–1039.
32 Mitniski AB, Mogilner AJ, Rockwood K: Accumulation of deficits as a proxy measure of aging. ScientificWorldJournal 2001;1:323–336.
33 Mitniski A, Xiaowei S, Skoog I, et al: Relative fitness and frailty in elderly men and women in developed countries and their relationship to mortality. J Am Geriatr Soc 2005;53:2184–2189.
34 Rockwood K, Andrew W, Mitniski A, et al: A comparison of two approaches measuring frailty in elderly people J Gerontol A Biol Sci Med Sci 2007;62:738–743.
35 Kulminski A, Ukraintseva SV, Akushevich IV, et al: Cumulative indices of health deficiencies as a characteristic of a long life. J Am Geriatr Soc 2007;55:935–940.
36 Goggins WB, Woo J, Sham A, et al: Frailty index as a measure of personal biological age in a Chinese population. J Gerontol A Biol Sci Med Sci 2005;60:1046–1051.
37 Searle SD, Mitniski A, Gahabauer EA, et al: A standard procedure for creating a frailty index. BMC Geriatr 2008;8:24–35.
38 Kamaruzzaman S, Ploubidis GB, Fletcher A, et al: A reliable measure of frailty for a community-dwelling older population. Health Qual Life Outcomes 2010;8:123–129.
39 Hastings SN, Purse JL, Johnson KS, et al: A frailty index predicts some but not all adverse outcomes in older adults discharged from the emergency department. J Am Geriatr Soc 2008;56:1651–1657.
40 Kulminski AM, Ukraintseva SV, Kulminskaya IV, et al: Cumulative deficits better characterize susceptibility to death in elderly than phenotypic frailty: lessons from the Cardiovascular Health Study. J Am Geriatr Soc 2008;56:898–903.
41 Rockwood K, Stadnyk K, MacKnight C, et al: a brief clinical instrument to classify frailty in elderly people. Lancet 1999;353:205–206.

42 Rockwood K, Song X, MacKnight C, et al: A global clinical measure of fitness and frailty in elderly people. CMAJ 2005;173:489–495.
43 Min L, Yoon W, Mariano J, et al: The Vulnerable Elder-13 Survey predicts 5-year functional decline and mortality outcome in older ambulatory care patients. J Am Geriatr Soc 2009;57:2070–2076.
44 Warshaw GA, Modawal A, Kues J, et al: Community physician education in geriatrics: applying the assessing care of the vulnerable elders model with a multisite primary care group. J Am Geriatr Soc 2010;58:1780–1785.
45 Reuben DB, Roth CP, Frank JC, et al: Assessing care of vulnerable elders Alzheimer's disease: a pilot study of a practice redesign intervention to improve the care of dementia. J Am Geriatr Soc 2010;58:324–329.
46 Anonymous: Assessing care of Vulnerable Elders-3 quality indicators. J Am Geriatr Soc 2007;55(suppl 2):S464–S487.

Lodovico Balducci, MD
Senior Adult Oncology Program
H. Lee Moffitt Cancer Center and Research Institute
University of South Florida
12902 Magnolia Drive, SA-Prog, Tampa, FL 33612 (USA)
E-Mail lodovico.balducci@moffitt.org

Targeting Age-Related Changes in the Biology of Acute Myeloid Leukemia: Is the Patient Seeing the Progress?

Norbert Vey

Institut Paoli-Calmettes and Aix-Marseille Université, Marseille, France

Abstract

The prognosis of acute myeloid leukemia (AML) in the elderly is poor with overall less than 5% of the patients expected to be alive after 5 years. In many studies, age was an independent poor prognostic factor. In the elderly, the frequency of secondary forms of AML, of unfavorable cytogenetics, expression of multidrug resistance genes in part explains the poor outcome. However, based on genetic and molecular studies, there is no evidence for specific biological features of the disease in the elderly. Host-related factors including comorbidity and reduced functional reserves also account for the severity of the disease. Finally, population-based studies show that approximately 30% of patients older than 65 years are offered intensive chemotherapy. This chapter summarizes the recent advances in the biology of AML, in particular the impact of new molecular markers. An overview of the studies that have evaluated comorbidities and results of geriatric assessments in these patients are also presented.

Copyright © 2013 S. Karger AG, Basel

Acute myeloid leukemia (AML) is the most common form of leukemia in adults. Its age-related incidence increases steeply after the age of 60 [1] and is about 75/100,000 in patients older than 75 [2]. Given the aging of the general population in Western countries, its incidence is expected to increase over time. Büchner et al. [3] recently reported that the proportion of patients older than 60 years included in the German AML Cooperative Group (AMLCG) went from 25% in the 1981 study to 53% in the 1999 study. This suggests that beyond quantitative changes, qualitative changes have also occurred, including improvement in the elderly health condition, willingness to receive intensive therapies, to participate in clinical trials. This also reflects societal changes and different views on what type of treatment elderly people want.

Since the 1970s, and thanks to the progress of intensive chemotherapy and allogeneic hematopoietic stem cell transplantation (SCT), AML is a curable disease. However, since most elderly patients cannot tolerate such therapeutic strategies and since they often present with chemoresistant diseases, their prognosis remains poor with few of them being cured. Appelbaum et al. [4] showed that over the 1973–1997 time period, unlike in younger patients, no improvement in survival was achieved in the elderly patients included in the consecutive ECOG trials. A similar observation was made from the results of MRC trials between 1970 and 2005 [5].

The development of successful therapeutic approaches in elderly patients with AML is thus a major challenge for hematologists. However, the recent advances in the understanding of the disease biology, the identification of new prognostic factors and the development of molecularly targeted therapies should contribute to improving treatments. In addition, the better understanding of the management of the oldest patients which have to be integrated into AML treatment strategies might also translate into substantial progress.

What Is AML?

AML is a clonal disease of hematopoietic stem cell which is characterized by a differentiation block, excessive self-renewal and proliferation, genetic instability, cell cycle deregulation, abnormal cell metabolism, adhesion or migration and resistance to apoptosis. According to the current model [6], the disease results from cooperation of type I mutations that affect proliferation (such as FLT3, RAS gene mutations) and type II mutations that affect differentiation (such as CEBPA, RUNX1 gene mutations). More recently, a third type of mutation has been described that affects epigenetic regulation (such as IDH1&2, DNMT3A). Some of these gene rearrangements are due to chromosome translocation, inversion or deletion and can be detected using conventional cytogenetics. The prognostic impact of cytogenetic categories has been clearly identified and used for treatment stratification in patients with AML and recently integrated in the WHO classification of myeloid neoplasms [7]. In addition, with the development of genomic technologies such as global gene expression analysis, next-generation sequencing and single nucleotide polymorphism (SNP) array analysis, a growing number of gene or gene expression abnormalities have been described including mutations of FLT3, NPM1, CEBPA, DNMT3A, IDH1&2, TET2 [for a review, see 8]. Based on this, the European Leukemia Net recently proposed a standardized reporting system for correlation of cytogenetic and molecular genetic data presented in table 1 [9] and risk-adjusted therapeutic strategies have been developed. For young patients, treatment intensity modulation according to risk, essentially rely on allogeneic SCT indications – a strategy which is associated with the highest relapse prevention potential offset by higher mortality risk. For instance, patients with t(8;21), inv(16) or t(16;16) or their molecular equivalents (also referred to as CBF-AMLs) have a favorable prognostic impact and are curable with high-dose cytarabine-including protocols. These patients are therefore no more considered candidates for allogeneic SCT in first CR. Recently,

Table 1. ELN genetic/molecular reporting system [9]

Genetic group	Subsets
Favorable	t(8;21)(q22;q22); *RUNX1-RUNX1T1* inv(16)(p13.1q22) or t(16;16)(p13.1;q22); *CBFB-MYH11* Mutated *NPM1* without *FLT3*-ITD (normal karyotype) Mutated *CEBPA* (normal karyotype)
Intermediate I	Mutated *NPM1* and *FLT3*-ITD (normal karyotype) Wild-type *NPM1* and *FLT3*-ITD (normal karyotype) Wild-type *NPM1* without *FLT3*-ITD (normal karyotype)
Intermediate II	t(9;11)(p22;q23); *MLLT3-MLL* Cytogenetic abnormalities not classified as favorable or adverse
Adverse	inv(3)(q21q26.2) or t(3;3)(q21;q26.2); *RPN1-EVI1* t(6;9)(p23;q34); *DEK-NUP214* t(v;11)(v;q23); *MLL* rearranged -5 or del(5q); -7; abnl(17p); complex karyotype

Schlenk et al. [10] showed that the patients who have no FLT3 mutation and have NPM1 or CEBPA mutation, have a comparable prognosis as those with CBF-AML and do not benefit from allogeneic SCT in first complete remission. Besides their critical role in risk-adjusted therapies, molecular alterations also represent targets for selected treatments such as anti-FLT3 kinase inhibitors [8] or all-*trans* retinoic acid for NPM1 mutated AMLs [11].

Biological Specificities of AML in the Elderly

Many factors concur to make AML in elderly a poor prognosis disease. Host-related factors are obvious explanations and are discussed below. Several differences in the disease biology have been described. They include:

(1) The frequency of forms arising from a preceding MDS which represent more than 20% of cases above the age of 60 [12] and are associated with resistance to chemotherapy.

(2) The frequency of multilineage dysplasia (which also reflects secondary forms to MDS and probably undiagnosed prior MDS). When assessed using 2008 WHO criteria, multilineage dysplasia was shown to increase in frequency with age and was associated with a poor outcome.

(3) Less proliferative disease reflected by lower median white blood cell (WBC) counts at diagnosis [3, 12] and fewer patients with hyperleukocytosis >20 g/l (40%

Table 2. Cytogenetic categories distribution in 1,435 elderly AML patients [data were pooled from 19–21]

Cytogenetic abnormality	Risk group	Number	Number by risk group
t(8;21)/inv(16)	favorable	62 (4%)	62 (4%)
Diploid	intermediate	606 (42%)	772 (53.5%)
Tri(8)	intermediate	166 (11.5%)	
Complex	unfavorable	219 (15%)	601 (41.5%)
-5/5q-	unfavorable	168 (11.5%)	
-7/7q-	unfavorable	180 (12.5%)	
11q23	unfavorable	34 (2%)	

vs. 50% in younger adults) [3]. One study also showed reduced LDH levels [3]. These differences are usually attributed to the increased frequency of secondary forms of AML in the elderly. However, lower WBC counts and LDH levels in the study of Büchner et al. [3] were observed after exclusion of secondary cases.

(4) An immature blast phenotype reflected by increased expression of CD34 and CD7 [13]. CD34 has been shown to predict poor CR rate in some studies [14] but not in all [15]. This effect might be related to association with MDR gene overexpression [16, 17] or to the fact that favorable prognosis NPM1 gene mutated AMLs do not express CD34 [18].

(5) The expression of drug resistance-associated genes such as MDR1, BRCP in increased in elderly patients [17]. Although conflicting data have been reported, the overexpression of these genes is considered as a poor prognostic feature in AML.

(6) A peculiar distribution of cytogenetic categories with less favorable cytogenetics (<5% vs. 20–25% in young adults). Table 2 presents the cytogenetic distribution in 1,289 elderly patients with AML who were included in three large multicenter trials all having received intensive induction chemotherapy [19–21].

Contrary to cytogenetic distribution, the frequency of the different gene mutations associated with a prognostic impact in young patients does not seem different. Specifically, FLT3 and NPM1 mutations frequency did not show age-related differences among patients with normal cytogenetics [3, 18]. In two CALBG series of elderly patients (>60 years) with normal karyotypes (169 and 243 patients), the frequency of other less frequent gene mutations such as CEBPA, IDH1, IDH2 or WT1 was in the range of that observed in younger patients [22, 23]. However, other studies showed conflicting results. Schneider et al. [24] reported that the proportion of patients with NPM1 mutations decreased after the age of 60 in their AMLSG series (40% NPM1 mutations in patients older than 60). This was also the case for FLT3

ITD (23% with FLT3-ITD) in that study and in another [24, 25]. On the other hand, in a recently published Chinese series, mutations of *NPM1*, *CEBPA* were more frequent in elderly patients [26]. Interestingly, this study also showed that nearly all of the genes regulating epigenetics tested (*DNMT3A*, *IDH1*, *IDH2*, and *TET2*, but not *MLL*) were also more frequently mutated in patients with higher median age.

Molecular epidemiology of AML in the elderly is still immature and explains the described discrepancies. However, the data suggests that there is no difference in the distribution of major gene mutations between younger and older patients. This observation does not support the hypothesis of intrinsic differences into the biology of AML in the elderly [3]. This has recently been confirmed by the comparison of the gene expression profile of NPM1 mutated AML between age groups which failed to show any difference [18].

It is thus likely that differences between young and old AML rely on the higher frequency of forms that arise from a previously recognized or not MDS as outlined by data from morphologic, phenotypic or cytogenetic analyses. For the other patients presenting with de novo AML, there is currently no data showing intrinsic biological age-related differences. Differences in patient outcome should thus be explained by differences in host-related factors and in the therapy.

Host-Disease Interactions in Elderly AML

Age is a major, if not the most important prognostic factor of AML and different therapeutic strategies are offered to patients younger or older than 60 years (a threshold that varies between 55 and 65 years in different AML cooperative groups) [9]. Even among the elderly population, age as a continuous variable is an independent prognostic factor [27, 28]. However, in the current practice, arbitrary age cut-offs are used and patients aged 75 and older are generally deemed not eligible for intensive treatments [28]. Age is in fact a surrogate for many patient-related covariates which include comorbidities, functional reserves, organ dysfunction. It is worth noting that AML differs from other cancers in that it often progresses rapidly, causes bone marrow failure which is responsible for infections, anemia and bleeding complications and can be associated with metabolic complications (renal dysfunction due tumor lysis syndrome) or involvement of organs (central nervous system, liver…). All these life-threatening complications can be responsible for rapid deterioration of the patients' general condition. It is therefore difficult to determine the respective role of the disease itself (reversible using anti-leukemic therapies) and of aging (essentially irreversible) in this deterioration at diagnosis [29]. For instance, a statistically significant association between high WBC counts (a marker of proliferative and therefore more aggressive forms of AML) and poor performance status (PS) was observed [27]. As a consequence, AML in the elderly is associated with a substantial rate of early deaths. Overall, large cooperative group studies of patients treated with

Table 3. Comorbidities evaluated using HCT-CI and revised HCT-CI

	Giles et al. [32]	Etienne et al. [14][1]	Malfuson et al. [27]	Harb et al. [33]	Savic et al. [34]
Patients, n	177	133	416	92	100
Median age (range)	70 (60–89)	73 (70–85)	72 (65–85)	83 (80–96)	69 (61–85)
HCT-CI					
0	22%	68%	25%	8%	29%
1–2	30%	29%	70%	33%	32%
≥3	48%	4%	5%	59%	39%
Prognostic value	CR/ED/OS	CR	OS	NA	ED/CR/OS

HCT-CI = Hematopoietic stem cell transplantation comorbidity index; CR = complete remission; ED = early death; OS = overall survival.
[1] Note that Sorror initial HCT-CI [36] was used while the revised version [35] was used in the other.

intensive chemotherapy show an early death rate of approximately 20% (as compared to 5% in younger patients) [9]. Death rates are also high in elderly patients who are not treated intensively: in a group of 93 elderly patients who received palliative chemotherapy or best supportive care at Institut Paoli-Calmettes, the median survival was 90 days [28]. Walter et al. [30] studied the kinetics of deaths in a large cohort of intensively treated patients and showed a peak in the risk of death within the first 4 weeks following diagnosis. In that study, age was a strong risk factor for early death, but other covariates such as PS, platelet counts, WBC counts, albumin, peripheral blast percentage, serum creatinine and secondary AML (yes/no) were also independent predictors of the 4-week treatment-related mortality (TRM). Interestingly, the model generated using these variables kept its predictive value for TRM even when age was withdrawn, indicating that age should be viewed as a surrogate for many other variables [30].

However, in that study as in others which evaluated prognostic factors in elderly AML [31], except for PS and creatinine, no parameters relating to the patients' comorbidities or functional alteration were analyzed. Available data regarding comorbidities in elderly AML patients are summarized in table 3 [14, 27, 32–34]. These studies used the hematopoietic stem cell transplantation comorbidity index (HCT-CI) which is an adaptation of the original Charlson Comorbidity Index developed in a large cohort of patients with hematologic malignancies (including 46% with AML). HCT-CI is predictive of TRM and survival after SCT [35, 36]. In these studies, different median age, selection criteria (cohorts of patients treated intensively or not) may explain inconsistencies in the distribution of the HCT-CI groups. In most of the studies however, only 25–30% of the patients had no comorbidity (score = 0) and cardiac disease represented the most frequent comorbidities. Interestingly, in one study [27], HCT-CI was shown to be independent from both age and PS, confirming previous results in solid tumors [37]. HCT-CI was correlated with various patient outcomes such as early death rate, complete remission achievement or overall survival (see table 3).

Little attention has been paid to other dimensions of vulnerability in AML patients. Notably, the use of Comprehensive Geriatric Assessment developed in elderly patients with cancers [38] has not yet been widely evaluated in AML. One study [39] evaluated prospectively instrumental activities of daily living as a marker of functional status impairment in a small series of AML from any age. Impairment of instrumental activities of daily living was predictive of survival. More recently, Klepin et al. [40] showed the feasibility of a Comprehensive Geriatric Assessment in a prospective study of 54 elderly AML patients (median age 70 years) among whom 63% had impairments of more than one functional domain. The impact of functional decline on patient outcome remains to be confirmed.

Treatment Options for Elderly Patients with AML

Intensive chemotherapy is the standard treatment for AML patients. It is based on combination of anthracyclines and cytarabine which are associated with CR rates of 50% and median overall survival of approximately 1 year [9]. A recent study of the HOVON group showed that intensified daunorubicin dose of 90 mg/m^2 was tolerable by elderly patients and was associated to better outcomes in the youngest old patients (60- to 65-year-old group) [41]. In general, attempts to intensify the postremission chemotherapy failed in this age group in most studies [42–45] but not all [46]. For a review, see Dombret et al. [47].

In a survey of the Surveillance, Epidemiology and End Results (SEER) US registry, only 30% of patients older than 65 years received intensive chemotherapy [48]. When compared to intensive chemotherapy, supportive care was inferior [49] while less intensive chemotherapy with low-dose cytarabine showed comparable CR duration and overall survival [50]. The issue for the clinicians is therefore to determine which patients will benefit from intensive approaches and which will not.

Currently, there is no effective nontoxic alternative therapy for the 'unfit' patients and this remains a field for clinical investigations. Among recently developed drugs, new cytotoxic agents such as clofarabine and laromustine, which produced CR rates of 32 and 28% respectively [51, 52] in patients not eligible for intensive chemotherapy, failed approval by regulation agencies both in Europe and in the USA. Demethylating agents have shown promising initial results [53, 54] which need confirmation in prospective randomized studies that are ongoing. The use of targeted therapies that are currently under investigation is attractive for the elderly AML population and might represent alternatives to conventional cytotoxic agents or be combined with chemotherapy. In addition, new forms of immunotherapy using WT1 vaccines or anti-KIR antibodies [55] are other promising approaches aiming at controlling post-chemotherapy residual disease.

How Can We Stratify Elderly Patients with AML?

The objective of any stratification system for elderly AML patients would be the accurate identification of those who could benefit from intensive chemotherapy. For those who could not, the alternative currently is the administration of palliative treatments (low-dose chemotherapy) with no expected impact on survival.

Cytogenetics remains the most significant prognostic factor for elderly AML. Different collaborative groups have developed classification systems. Basically, the favorable group is comprised of patients with inv(16) or t(8;21) (except for the AMLSG [20]), unfavorable of patients with complex cytogenetics, and the intermediate group of patients with normal or other karyotypes [19–21, 56]. Continuing analyses of large cytogenetic database allow for improvement of cytogenetic classifications. Recently, autosomal monosomy (i.e. one autosomal monosomy associated with another monosomy or one structural abnormality seen in less than 10% of adults) was associated with an extremely poor prognosis (4-year OS = 4%) [57, 58].

The use of new molecular markers might improve prognostication, especially in the group with normal cytogenetics. The prognostic impact of NPM1 and FLT3 mutations is retained in elderly patients when analyzed independently [18, 23] or in combination [3]. NPM1 mutations were associated with improved CR rate, relapse-free and overall survival [3, 18] while the unfavorable impact of FLT3-ITD was on overall and disease-free survival only [23]. In another series of 158 elderly patients with normal cytogenetics who received intensive chemotherapy, NPM1 mutations impacted the CR rate but not overall survival, while FLT3-ITD impacted only disease-free survival by multivariate analysis [22]. The same study found low expression of ERG and BAAL-C genes to be associated with a favorable outcome [22].

When using cytogenetic or molecular risk stratification models, it should be kept in mind that in each category, the outcome of elderly patients is worse than that of younger patients in the same category [3]. This is illustrated by the results of the French Intergroup study of elderly patients with CBF-AMLs which showed that, although considered as 'favorable', 2-year overall survival in that group was only 27% [59].

Patient-related risk factors have a prognostic impact independent from that of cytogenetic or molecular factors. They include PS, WBC counts, LDH levels and serum creatinine levels. In addition, use of comorbidity scoring with HCT-CI was shown to predict patient outcome in five studies shown in table 3 [14, 27, 32–34].

Several groups have proposed prognostic models aiming at helping in treatment decision-making. It is worth noting that the proposed scoring systems were generated

Table 4. Prognostic models for elderly AML patients

	Endpoint	Variables	High-risk group		
			criteria	% of HR patients	outcome of HR patients
Malfuson et al. [27]	D100 mortality	unfavorable K age >75 PS ≥2 WBC ≥50 g/l	unfavorable K or ≥2 other factors	24%	19% 1-year OS
Kantarjian et al. [31]	8-week mortality	age >80 years complex K PS >1 creatinine >1.3	>3 factors	9%	8-week mortality = 71%
Etienne et al. [14]	CR	WBC ≥30 g/l CD34+ HCT-CI >1 unfavorable K	score >2	37%	8-week mortality = 34% 2-year OS = 15%

HCT-CI = Hematopoietic stem cell transplantation comorbidity index; CR = complete remission; OS = overall survival; HR = high-risk; K = karyotype.

from databases which included elderly patients treated with intensive chemotherapy who represent only 30–45% of patients older than 65 years diagnosed with AML [48]. This selection bias represents an obvious limitation to the conclusions of these studies and explains the relatively low proportion of patients with high comorbidity scores in these series [14, 27, 32–34]. Different prognostic models have thus been proposed with the objective of identifying the subset of patients who do not benefit from the use of intensive chemotherapy [14, 27, 31]. Despite the differences in variables, endpoints and methods used in these studies which are presented in table 4, these models identify a group of patients representing 30–40% of the entire population who have an early mortality rate (defined as 8-week mortality) higher than 30%.

Have the Patients Seen the Progress?

The answer is no, since the overall survival of elderly patients with AML remains extremely poor, since intensive chemotherapy is at yet the only active approach which can be offered to less than 40% of the patients, and since there are no established criteria for the definition of the patient population likely to benefit from intensive chemotherapy. However, the use of molecular markers together with the use of geriatric assessment might help in refining the current prognostic models and improve their accuracy.

In addition, new therapies currently being developed for the treatment of AML include many drugs with a low toxicity profile which could be given to elderly patients. 926 clinical trials including AML patients older than 65 are currently registered at ClinicalTrials.gov, reflecting the interest and new possibilities for this group of patients.

The patients might soon see the progress...

References

1 Xie Y, Davies SM, Xiang Y, et al: Trends in leukemia incidence and survival in the United States (1973–1998). Cancer 2003;97:2229–2235.
2 Howlader N: SEER Cancer Statistics Review 1975–2008. 2010.
3 Büchner T, Berdel WE, Haferlach C, et al: Age-related risk profile and chemotherapy dose response in acute myeloid leukemia: a study by the German Acute Myeloid Leukemia Cooperative Group. J Clin Oncol 2009;27:61–69.
4 Appelbaum FR, Rowe JM, Radich J, Dick JE: Acute myeloid leukemia. Hematology Am Soc Hematol Educ Program 2001;2001:62–86.
5 Burnett AK, Mohite U: Treatment of older patients with acute myeloid leukemia – new agents. Semin Hematol 2006;43:96–106.
6 Gilliland DG, Griffin JD: The roles of FLT3 in hematopoiesis and leukemia. Blood 2002;100:1532–1542.
7 Vardiman JW, Thiele J, Arber DA, et al: The 2008 revision of the World Health Organization (WHO) classification of myeloid neoplasms and acute leukemia: rationale and important changes. Blood 2009;114:937–951.
8 Dohner H, Gaidzik VI: Impact of genetic features on treatment decisions in AML. Hematology Am Soc Hematol Educ Program 2011;2011:36–42.
9 Dohner H, Estey EH, Amadori S, et al: Diagnosis and management of acute myeloid leukemia in adults: recommendations from an international expert panel, on behalf of the European LeukemiaNet. Blood 2010;115:453–474.
10 Schlenk RF, Dohner K, Krauter J, et al: Mutations and treatment outcome in cytogenetically normal acute myeloid leukemia. N Engl J Med 2008;358:1909–1918.
11 Schlenk RF, Dohner K, Kneba M, et al: Gene mutations and response to treatment with all-*trans* retinoic acid in elderly patients with acute myeloid leukemia. Results from the AMLSG Trial AML HD98B. Haematologica 2009;94:54–60.
12 Appelbaum FR, Gundacker H, Head DR, et al: Age and acute myeloid leukemia. Blood 2006;107:3481–3485.
13 Leith CP, Kopecky KJ, Godwin J, et al: Acute myeloid leukemia in the elderly: assessment of multidrug resistance (MDR1) and cytogenetics distinguishes biologic subgroups with remarkably distinct responses to standard chemotherapy. A Southwest Oncology Group Study. Blood 1997;89:3323–3329.
14 Etienne A, Esterni B, Charbonnier A, et al: Comorbidity is an independent predictor of complete remission in elderly patients receiving induction chemotherapy for acute myeloid leukemia. Cancer 2007;109:1376–1383.
15 Pinto A, Zagonel V, Ferrara F: Acute myeloid leukemia in the elderly: biology and therapeutic strategies. Crit Rev Oncol Hematol 2001;39:275–287.
16 List AF, Spier CM, Cline A, et al: Expression of the multidrug resistance gene product (P-glycoprotein) in myelodysplasia is associated with a stem cell phenotype. Br J Haematol 1991;78:28–34.
17 Van den Heuvel-Eibrink MM, van der Holt B, Burnett AK, et al: CD34-related coexpression of MDR1 and BCRP indicates a clinically resistant phenotype in patients with acute myeloid leukemia of older age. Ann Hematol 2007;86:329–337.
18 Becker H, Marcucci G, Maharry K, et al: Favorable prognostic impact of NPM1 mutations in older patients with cytogenetically normal de novo acute myeloid leukemia and associated gene- and microRNA-expression signatures: a Cancer and Leukemia Group B Study. J Clin Oncol 2010;28:596–604.
19 Farag SS, Archer KJ, Mrozek K, et al: Pretreatment cytogenetics add to other prognostic factors predicting complete remission and long-term outcome in patients 60 years of age or older with acute myeloid leukemia: results from Cancer and Leukemia Group B 8461. Blood 2006;108:63–73.
20 Frohling S, Schlenk RF, Kayser S, et al: Cytogenetics and age are major determinants of outcome in intensively treated acute myeloid leukemia patients older than 60 years: results from AMLSG trial AML HD98-B. Blood 2006;108:3280–3288.

21 Van der Holt B, Breems DA, Berna Beverloo H, et al: Various distinctive cytogenetic abnormalities in patients with acute myeloid leukaemia aged 60 years and older express adverse prognostic value: results from a prospective clinical trial. Br J Haematol 2007;136:96–105.

22 Schwind S, Marcucci G, Maharry K, et al: BAALC and ERG expression levels are associated with outcome and distinct gene and microRNA expression profiles in older patients with de novo cytogenetically normal acute myeloid leukemia: a Cancer and Leukemia Group B Study. Blood 2010;116:5660–5669.

23 Whitman SP, Maharry K, Radmacher MD, et al: FLT3 internal tandem duplication associates with adverse outcome and gene- and microRNA-expression signatures in patients 60 years of age or older with primary cytogenetically normal acute myeloid leukemia: a Cancer and Leukemia Group B Study. Blood 2010;116:3622–3626.

24 Schneider F, Hoster E, Schneider S, et al: Age-dependent frequencies of NPM1 mutations and FLT3-ITD in patients with normal karyotype AML (NK-AML). Ann Hematol 2012;91:9–18.

25 Schnittger S, Schoch C, Dugas M, et al: Analysis of FLT3 length mutations in 1,003 patients with acute myeloid leukemia: correlation to cytogenetics, FAB subtype, and prognosis in the AMLCG study and usefulness as a marker for the detection of minimal residual disease. Blood 2002;100:59–66.

26 Shen Y, Zhu YM, Fan X, et al: Gene mutation patterns and their prognostic impact in a cohort of 1,185 patients with acute myeloid leukemia. Blood 2011;118:5593–5603.

27 Malfuson JV, Etienne A, Turlure P, et al: Risk factors and decision criteria for intensive chemotherapy in older patients with acute myeloid leukemia. Haematologica 2008;93:1806–1813.

28 Vey N, Coso D, Bardou VJ, et al: The benefit of induction chemotherapy in patients age > or = 75 years. Cancer 2004;101:325–331.

29 Ferrara F: Treatment of unfit patients with acute myeloid leukemia: a still open clinical challenge. Clin Lymphoma Myeloma Leuk 2011;11:10–16.

30 Walter RB, Othus M, Borthakur G, et al: Prediction of early death after induction therapy for newly diagnosed acute myeloid leukemia with pretreatment risk scores: a novel paradigm for treatment assignment. J Clin Oncol 2011;29:4417–4423.

31 Kantarjian H, Ravandi F, O'Brien S, et al: Intensive chemotherapy does not benefit most older patients (age 70 years or older) with acute myeloid leukemia. Blood 2010;116:4422–4429.

32 Giles FJ, Borthakur G, Ravandi F, et al: The haematopoietic cell transplantation comorbidity index score is predictive of early death and survival in patients over 60 years of age receiving induction therapy for acute myeloid leukaemia. Br J Haematol 2007;136:624–627.

33 Harb AJ, Tan W, Wilding GE, et al: Treating octogenarian and nonagenarian acute myeloid leukemia patients – predictive prognostic models. Cancer 2009;115:2472–2481.

34 Savic A, Kvrgic V, Rajic N, et al: The hematopoietic cell transplantation comorbidity index is a predictor of early death and survival in adult acute myeloid leukemia patients. Leuk Res 2012;36:479–482.

35 Sorror ML, Maris MB, Storb R, et al: Hematopoietic cell transplantation (HCT)-specific comorbidity index: a new tool for risk assessment before allogeneic HCT. Blood 2005;106:2912–2919.

36 Sorror ML, Maris MB, Storer B, et al: Comparing morbidity and mortality of HLA-matched unrelated donor hematopoietic cell transplantation after nonmyeloablative and myeloablative conditioning: influence of pretransplantation comorbidities. Blood 2004;104:961–968.

37 Extermann M, Overcash J, Lyman GH, et al: Comorbidity and functional status are independent in older cancer patients. J Clin Oncol 1998;16:1582–1587.

38 Extermann M, Hurria A: Comprehensive geriatric assessment for older patients with cancer. J Clin Oncol 2007;25:1824–1831.

39 Wedding U, Rohrig B, Klippstein A, et al: Impairment in functional status and survival in patients with acute myeloid leukaemia. J Cancer Res Clin Oncol 2006;132:665–671.

40 Klepin HD, Geiger AM, Tooze JA, et al: The feasibility of inpatient geriatric assessment for older adults receiving induction chemotherapy for acute myelogenous leukemia. J Am Geriatr Soc 2011;59:1837–1846.

41 Lowenberg B, Ossenkoppele GJ, van Putten W, et al: High-dose daunorubicin in older patients with acute myeloid leukemia. N Engl J Med 2009;361:1235–1248.

42 Buchner T, Hiddemann W, Berdel WE, et al: 6-Thioguanine, cytarabine, and daunorubicin (TAD) and high-dose cytarabine and mitoxantrone (HAM) for induction, TAD for consolidation, and either prolonged maintenance by reduced monthly TAD or TAD-HAM-TAD and one course of intensive consolidation by sequential HAM in adult patients at all ages with de novo acute myeloid leukemia (AML): a randomized trial of the German AML Cooperative Group. J Clin Oncol 2003;21:4496–4504.

43 Gardin C, Turlure P, Fagot T, et al: Postremission treatment of elderly patients with acute myeloid leukemia in first complete remission after intensive induction chemotherapy: results of the multicenter randomized Acute Leukemia French Association (ALFA) 9803 trial. Blood 2007;109:5129–5135.

44 Goldstone AH, Burnett AK, Wheatley K, et al: Attempts to improve treatment outcomes in acute myeloid leukemia in older patients: the results of the United Kingdom Medical Research Council AML11 trial. Blood 2001;98:1302–1311.

45 Stone RM, Berg DT, George SL, et al: Postremission therapy in older patients with de novo acute myeloid leukemia: a randomized trial comparing mitoxantrone and intermediate-dose cytarabine with standard-dose cytarabine. Blood 2001;98:548–553.

46 Schlenk RF, Frohling S, Hartmann F, et al: Intensive consolidation versus oral maintenance therapy in patients 61 years or older with acute myeloid leukemia in first remission: results of second randomization of the AML HD98-B Treatment Trial. Leukemia 2006;20:748–750.

47 Dombret H, Raffoux E, Gardin C: Acute myeloid leukemia in the elderly. Semin Oncol 2008;35:430–438.

48 Menzin J, Lang K, Earle CC, et al: The outcomes and costs of acute myeloid leukemia among the elderly. Arch Intern Med 2002;162:1597–1603.

49 Lowenberg B, Zittoun R, Kerkhofs H, et al: On the value of intensive remission-induction chemotherapy in elderly patients of 65+ years with acute myeloid leukemia: a randomized phase III study of the European Organization for Research and Treatment of Cancer Leukemia Group. J Clin Oncol 1989;7:1268–1274.

50 Tilly H, Castaigne S, Bordessoule D, et al: Low-dose cytarabine versus intensive chemotherapy in the treatment of acute nonlymphocytic leukemia in the elderly. J Clin Oncol 1990;8:272–279.

51 Burnett AK, Russell NH, Kell J, et al: European development of clofarabine as treatment for older patients with acute myeloid leukemia considered unsuitable for intensive chemotherapy. J Clin Oncol 2010;28:2389–2395.

52 Giles F, Rizzieri D, Karp J, et al: Cloretazine (VNP40101M), a novel sulfonylhydrazine alkylating agent, in patients age 60 years or older with previously untreated acute myeloid leukemia. J Clin Oncol 2007;25:25–31.

53 Cashen AF, Schiller GJ, O'Donnell MR, DiPersio JF: Multicenter, phase II study of decitabine for the first-line treatment of older patients with acute myeloid leukemia. J Clin Oncol 2010;28:556–561.

54 Fenaux P, Mufti GJ, Hellstrom-Lindberg E, et al: Azacitidine prolongs overall survival compared with conventional care regimens in elderly patients with low bone marrow blast count acute myeloid leukemia. J Clin Oncol 2010;28:562–569.

55 Vey N, Bourhis J, Dombret H, et al: A phase I study of the anti-natural killer inhibitory receptor monoclonal antibody (1-7F9, IPH2101) in elderly patients with acute myeloid leukemia. J Clin Oncol 2009; 27(suppl), abstr 3015.

56 Grimwade D, Walker H, Harrison G, et al: The predictive value of hierarchical cytogenetic classification in older adults with acute myeloid leukemia: analysis of 1,065 patients entered into the United Kingdom Medical Research Council AML11 Trial. Blood 2001;98:1312–1320.

57 Breems DA, Van Putten WL, De Greef GE, et al: Monosomal karyotype in acute myeloid leukemia: a better indicator of poor prognosis than a complex karyotype. J Clin Oncol 2008;26:4791–4797.

58 Perrot A, Luquet I, Pigneux A, et al: Dismal prognostic value of monosomal karyotype in elderly patients with acute myeloid leukemia: a GOELAMS study of 186 patients with unfavorable cytogenetic abnormalities. Blood 2011;118:679–685.

59 Prebet T, Boissel N, Reutenauer S, et al: Acute myeloid leukemia with translocation (8;21) or inversion (16) in elderly patients treated with conventional chemotherapy: a collaborative study of the French CBF-AML intergroup. J Clin Oncol 2009;27:4747–4753.

Prof. Norbert Vey, MD
Institut Paoli-Calmettes
232, Blvd. de Sainte Marguerite
FR–13008 Marseille (France)
E-Mail veyn@marseille.fnclcc.fr

Comprehensive Geriatric Assessment in Oncology

Supriya G. Mohile · Allison Magnuson

School of Medicine and Dentistry, University of Rochester Medical Center, Rochester, N.Y., USA

Abstract

The incidence of cancer increases with advanced age and the majority of cancer deaths are in patients aged ≥65. The geriatric population is a heterogeneous group and a patient's chronologic age does not always correlate with underlying physiologic status. Oncologists need to be able to obtain information on physiologic and functional capacity in older patients in order to provide safe and effective treatment recommendations. The Comprehensive Geriatric Assessment (CGA) is a compilation of validated tools that predict morbidity and mortality in community-dwelling older adults. The various components of the CGA have also been shown to influence clinical decision-making and predict outcomes in older cancer patients. The combined data from the CGA can be used to stratify patients into risk categories to better predict their tolerance to treatment and risk for chemotherapy toxicity. However, the CGA is a comprehensive tool requiring significant time and training to perform. A variety of screening tools have been developed which may be useful in the general oncology practice setting to identify patients that may benefit from further testing and intervention. This chapter will review the components and predictive value of CGA in older cancer patients, with emphasis on how CGA can practically be incorporated into clinical practice.

Copyright © 2013 S. Karger AG, Basel

Older patients commonly have health status issues that can affect cancer outcomes. For example, up to 50% of cancer patients require assistance with independent activities of daily living, which measure the ability for an older person to complete tasks necessary to live independently in the community [1]. Additionally, one quarter of patients have some form of cognitive impairment which can impact cancer-related outcomes [2]. The Comprehensive Geriatric Assessment (CGA) is an evaluation tool utilized by geriatricians to assess overall health status. The CGA includes validated tools of functional status, comorbidities, cognition, social support system, nutrition and medication review. In community-dwelling older adults, impairments in these domains predict morbidity and mortality. In cancer patients, measures within geriatric assessment can predict postoperative morbidity, toxicity of chemotherapy, and mortality [1]. CGA can aid oncologists in predicting outcomes and selecting appropriate treatment regimens and interventions for their patients. However, it is a comprehensive tool requiring significant time and manpower to adequately perform, and may not be practical for the general oncologist in the outpatient setting. Therefore, a variety of screening tools which aim to assess patients for potential areas of impairment are being researched.

In this chapter, we will provide an overview of the components of the CGA. We will provide information on validated tools that can help identify impairments in geriatric domains within the CGA and also describe the predictive value of each of these tools in identifying vulnerability in older adults with cancer. We will also provide practical considerations on how to utilize CGA in clinical practice to inform decision-making for treatment, identify those patients most likely to develop chemotherapy toxicity, and to guide interventions to improve outcomes.

Components of Geriatric Assessment (table 1)

Functional Status
Traditionally, oncologists have used performance status (i.e., ECOG or Karnofsky performance status scales) as an assessment of functional status. Poor performance on the ECOG scale has been associated with decreased survival in older patients being treated with palliative chemotherapy for advanced cancer [3, 4]. Functional assessment using oncology performance status measures alone, however, is inadequate when determining risk for many older adults with cancer. Scores of 0–2 encompass a broad range of functions in older adults. Many older patients present with an ECOG score of <3 in clinical practice [5]. Extermann and Hurria [1] demonstrated that although only 20% of geriatric oncology patients present with a performance status of ≥2, more than half of this population needs assistance with instrumental activities of daily living (IADLs), which measure the ability of a person to perform tasks that allow for living independently in the community (e.g., shopping, managing money). Repetto et al. [5] studied 363 elderly cancer patients and found that of those with good performance status, 37.7% had IADL limitations.

In geriatrics, functional status is commonly assessed using activities of daily living (ADL) and IADL scales [6, 7]. ADLs are skills required for basic self-care, such as the ability to bathe, feed, dress, toilet and transfer oneself as well as maintain continence [6]. These skills are necessary to maintain independence in one's own home whereas IADLs are the skills necessary to maintain independence in the community. IADLs include the ability to perform housekeeping and laundry, meal preparation and grocery shopping, medication administration, finance management, ability to access transportation systems, and use the telephone [7]. These task-specific scales have been proposed for use in a geriatric assessment for older cancer patients, since they add vital information to the ECOG and Karnofsky performance scales. Dependence

Table 1. CGA domains and measurement options

Domains	Definition	Measurement options
Function/ physical performance	– Ability to take care of one's self-care needs to live independently at home – Ability to care for tasks that allow independence in the community – Physical performance is an objective evaluation of mobility, balance, and fall risk	Activities of daily living Instrumental activities of daily living History of falls Timed up and go Short Physical Performance Battery Handgrip testing
Comorbidity/ pharmacy	– Chronic diseases that influence life expectancy and may influence tolerance to cancer treatment – Medications can increase risk of adverse events with cancer treatment	Charlson Comorbidity Scale Cumulative Illness Rating Scale-Geriatrics Comorbidity count and severity Medication Count Beers Criteria
Cognition	– Common in older patients and may affect decision-making capacity and interfere with cancer treatment	Mini-Mental Status Examination Blessed Orientation Memory Scale Short Portable Mental Status Questionnaire Montreal Cognitive Assessment
Psychological status	– Depression and anxiety are independently associated with adverse outcomes in cancer patients	Geriatric Depression Scale Hospital Anxiety and Depression Scale
Nutrition	– Weight loss and anorexia affect tolerance to treatment and survival in older cancer patients	Mini-Nutritional Assessment Weight loss Body mass index
Social support	– Adequate social support necessary for older patients to successfully undergo treatment	Needs assessment of financial capabilities, transportation, and caregiver status Medical Outcomes Survey Social Support

on others for ADL and IADL assistance has been shown to be predictive of mortality in geriatric oncology patients [8] and it has been observed that older patients with cancer have a higher incidence of ADL and IADL deficiencies when compared to age-matched controls [9].

In studies of geriatric assessment of older patients with cancer, a substantial number presented with ADL or IADL disabilities [10–12]. For example, Girre et al. [11] evaluated 105 patients aged ≥70 with breast cancer, and reported that 42% required assistance with ADLs and 54% required assistance with IADLs, despite the fact that only 7% of patients received an ECOG score >2. A significant proportion (>40%) of patients had functional deficits as measured by IADLs in two large studies developed to examine factors that predict chemotherapy toxicity [13, 14]. Predictive models for chemotherapy toxicity and survival are discussed later in the chapter. At the time of this review, there is no consensus regarding how to modify treatment plans according to underlying functional status and more studies are needed to evaluate the safety and efficacy of standard treatment approaches for cancer in patients with baseline IADL deficits.

Objective Physical Performance
Physical performance measures are standardized objective measures that provide a quantitative and reproducible assessment of specific functional tasks such as walking speed, lower extremity strength, or grip strength. These tests complement self-report functional assessment by detecting subclinical changes that may also predict morbidity and mortality. Objective physical performance measures have been shown to predict hospitalizations, disability, and mortality in the ambulatory geriatric population [15, 16]. These measures include the Short Physical Performance Battery (SPPB) and the 'Timed Get Up and Go' test, and isometric grip strength [15–17]. The SPPB measures balance, chair stands (strength), and gait speed. This tool has been validated in community-dwelling older adults and is highly predictive of future disability, nursing home placement, and mortality [18]. Although the predictive value of the SPPB for predicting adverse outcomes in older cancer patients is yet unknown, specific populations of older cancer patients have been shown to have significant issues with physical performance as measured by the SPPB. For example, in a study of 50 older men with prostate cancer on androgen deprivation therapy, 56% had abnormal SPPB findings and deficits occurred within all subcomponents (balance, walking, and chair stands) [19]. The Timed Get Up and Go test has been evaluated as part of a geriatric assessment in older cancer patients and has been shown to be feasible in both the clinical and cooperative (clinical trial) group setting [20]. This test measures how many seconds it takes an individual to stand from a seated position, walk a distance of 10 ft, turn, walk back to the chair and sit down again [17]. The simplicity of this test makes it a practical choice for the clinical setting.

Consensus guidelines, including the NCCN, do recommend physical performance assessments in addition to oncology performance scales in making decisions about treatment [21–23]. Future prospective studies will help to validate these measures and provide clinical cutoff scores to be used in different clinical settings.

Comorbidity
The relative incidence of comorbid conditions increases with age. This holds true for cancer patients as well. Yancik [24] evaluated 7,600 patients with cancer and found that those aged ≥75 years had an average of 4.2 comorbid conditions, whereas those <75 years had an average of 2.9 comorbid conditions. Several studies have shown

similar associations between the presence of comorbid conditions and prognosis in older cancer patients [25–28].

Comorbid conditions may affect a patient's toxicity risk from treatment for their cancer. In a study by Wildes et al. [29], 152 patients who underwent BEAM conditioning followed by autologous stem cell transplantation were studied to evaluate the impact of comorbidity on toxicity and mortality. Comorbid conditions, as assessed by the Charlson Comorbidity Index, significantly correlated with treatment-related mortality. Several studies have reported that hormonal treatment (i.e., androgen deprivation therapy) is associated with increased mortality in patients with underlying heart disease [30, 31]. In a randomized adjuvant chemotherapy trial of patients with high-risk stage II and III colon cancer, those with diabetes mellitus experienced a significantly higher rate of overall mortality and cancer recurrence [32]. One nationally representative population-based study reported a significantly higher number of comorbidities in cancer survivors compared to those without cancer [33].

Analysis of a patient's life expectancy from comorbid conditions versus the malignancy-related mortality must be considered when evaluating treatment options. If an alternative comorbid condition portends a shorter survival time than expected from the malignancy, the risks of cancer therapy could outweigh the benefit. Life expectancy can be obtained from life expectancy tables published by multiple national organizations [34] and from Walters et al. [35].

Polypharmacy
Age-related changes in physiology can influence the pharmacodynamics and pharmacokinetics of cancer-related drugs, thus affecting the efficacy as well as toxicity [36, 37]. Predicting drug efficacy and tolerance is even more complicated because of the high prevalence of polypharmacy in this population [38, 39]. The prevalence of polypharmacy in the elderly ranges widely and depends on the population studied as well as the definition of polypharmacy used. In studies evaluating community-dwelling individuals over the age of 65 in the ambulatory care setting, the prevalence of polypharmacy ranged between 15.6 and 94.3% [40–43]. Studies of older adults with cancer report the average number of medications ranges from 4 to 9, depending on the population sampled [38, 39, 44, 45].

Polypharmacy is associated with adverse drug reactions, increased risk of drug-drug interactions, and decreased compliance with medications [38]. These risks are particularly important considerations in older adults who are challenged with chemotherapy treatments. There are no evidence-based guidelines for evaluation and management of polypharmacy in older cancer patients. The Beers Criteria identifies specific drugs or drug classes which may have increased side effect profiles in older patients in general, particularly when a safer alternative drug option exists [46]. It is also important to assess a patient's non-prescription medication, including all herbals and supplements. Recent studies suggest the prevalence of complimentary/alternative medication use in the elderly population is 26–36% [47, 48]. Herbal supplements increase the risk for drug interactions and may affect clearance rates of chemotherapy [49]. Studies have shown that incorporating a pharmacist into clinical care decreases suboptimal prescribing and potentially lead to a decrease of adverse drug events [42, 50–52].

Cognition
One fifth of geriatric cancer patients screened positively for cognitive disorders in an academic setting [53, 54]. The prevalence of dementia increases to 25–48% in samples of community-living populations over 80 years of age [55]. The prevalence of early or mild cognitive impairment is estimated to be even higher [55, 56]. Cognitive impairment is associated with an increased risk for progression to dementia, with progression rates of 10–15% per year as compared with 1–2.5% in persons who are cognitively intact [56–58]. Cognitive disorders such as dementia limit life expectancy [59].

Cognitive impairments in geriatric patients with cancer often are under-recognized and undiagnosed. Patients with mild cognitive impairment are often more difficult to identify and deficits may only be recognized on cognitive assessment. In studies of patients undergoing CGA, approximately 20% of patients screen positive for some degree of cognitive disorder [24, 60]. The presence of cognitive disorders, particularly more advanced disease, may limit life expectancy [59] and influence the decision to institute cancer-related treatment. The diagnosis of dementia can have major impact on cancer diagnosis and treatment patterns [61–63]. The presence of cognitive disorders affects compliance to medications, consent to treatment, and caregiver burden. Cognitive impairment has been shown to affect cancer treatment with impaired persons receiving less definitive cancer care than other patients [61, 63, 64]. For example, a population-based study of patients with colon cancer and comorbid dementia found that patients with dementia were less likely to receive definitive treatment and that many did not even undergo initial diagnostic procedures [61]. Additionally, patients with cognitive disorders may have a higher risk of treatment toxicity and hospitalizations due to having more difficulty with following complex instructions, taking medications, and reporting treatment-related side effects.

Over the last several years, investigators have prospectively studied the impact of cancer treatment on cognitive functioning following up on patients' complaints of changes in memory and concentration. In one longitudinal prospective study of older patients with breast cancer, 51% of 45 evaluable patients perceived a decline in cognitive function after 6 months of chemotherapy [65]. Other studies demonstrated no significant change in Mini-Mental Status Examination (MMSE) scores after chemotherapy or hormonal therapy over a short period of time [10, 66]. Although more prospective, long-term, larger studies are necessary to elucidate the true impact of cancer treatment on the cognitive function, one population-based study suggests that women with breast cancer who receive chemotherapy have a higher likelihood of developing a dementia diagnosis after long-term follow-up [62]. Clinical trials and observational studies should consider including measures of cognitive functioning to examine the impact of cancer treatment longitudinally.

A cognitive assessment tool within the CGA for older cancer patients should be able to screen for baseline impairment and potentially follow effects of therapy on cognitive functioning. Clinical suspicion of dementia is not as sensitive as available screening tools [67]. Cognitive screening tools that have been studied include the Blessed Dementia Rating Scale [68], MMSE [69] Mini-Cog [70], and Short Portable Mental Status Questionnaire [71]. The purpose of screening is to assess cognitive capacity and to stratify risk. Abnormal scores on screening tools should trigger a comprehensive work-up with cognitive specialists. These tools have not yet demonstrated sufficient ability to detect changes in cognition that may be due to treatment, and a more detailed neuropsychological evaluation may be needed to accomplish this goal [65].

Nutrition

Nutritional status is in important prognostic indicator in the geriatric population. Weight loss is a marker for declining nutritional status and often observed in the geriatric population, particularly in those who are frail. Weight loss is one of the criteria for frailty as developed through the Cardiovascular Health Study, which established the phenotype of frailty in community-dwelling older adults [72]. In the non-cancer population, studies of community-dwelling geriatric patients found a twofold increased risk of mortality in those patients with a weight loss of 5% body weight [73]. In the cancer population, weight loss [74] and malnutrition [4] prior to diagnosis have been associated with worse overall survival rates.

A variety of screening tools are available to identify malnutrition. These tools include self-reported weight loss, calculation of body mass index (BMI) with BMI ≤20 associated with adverse outcomes, and the Mini-Nutritional Assessment (MNA). The MNA has been validated in the geriatric population and includes anthropometric measurements as well as questions related to diet and lifestyle, self-perceived health, mobility and medications. It has been shown to be a sensitive and specific tool for identifying malnutrition in the elderly population as well as recognizing those patients at higher risk for malnutrition [75].

Social Support and Financial Considerations

Consideration of a patient's social support network is an important component of a CGA. In both geriatric and oncology literature, social isolation has been associated with increased risk of mortality [76, 77]. Cancer patients, in general, require considerable support from a caregiver. They often require assistance with transportation for treatment sessions and support with symptom management if they experience side effects from their therapy. A study by Osborne et al. [78] evaluated a retrospective cohort of breast cancer patients using linked Medicare and SEER cancer registry data. The sample included 32,268 women, aged 65 and older. They found that unmarried women were more likely to be diagnosed with advanced stage cancer as compared to married women. Additionally, they were less likely to receive definitive care for their disease and more likely to die from their breast cancer.

Social support may be assessed in a variety of ways [79]. The most commonly used method to evaluate social support within a CGA is the Medical Outcomes Study Social Support Survey. This is a survey of 20 items assessing a patient's perceived availability of social support. Additionally, the impact of overall health on social functioning is important to assess, given the increased association with mortality in patient with social isolation. This is often measured using the Medical Outcomes Study Social Activity Limitations Measure, which is 4-item questionnaire evaluating the extent that a patient's physical or emotional problems interfere with their social activities.

Cancer care is expensive [80]. Older patients with Medicare face significant 'out-of-pocket' cancer costs [81, 82]. Many gaps exist within Medicare coverage for healthcare including private nursing, physical therapy or rehabilitation, transportation, dental care, eyeglasses, and hearing aids. These services are often inherently necessary for adequate cancer care and can be prohibitively expensive for some elderly. Many elderly persons must pay for their medications out-of-pocket because prescription drug coverage including those drugs needed for supportive care like pain management and nausea control are not always fully covered. The copayments for newer oral targeted therapies can be prohibitively expensive. As a result, seniors with limited fixed incomes may forgo supportive medications such as anti-nausea or pain medications if faced with a decision of affording either an anti-cancer drug or the adjunctive supportive medications [80].

Evaluation of social support and financial barriers in older adults with cancer is essential as it informs providers of strategies for appropriate care and should allow for early recognition of potential problems/needs of the patient with initiation of preventative intervention measures [83]. A social worker with a background in aging should be involved in the assessment of an older patient in order to identify community and financial resources that could help meet the patient's needs.

Psychological Distress

Older adults with cancer reportedly experience similar or less distress than younger adults [84]. Distress is defined as a 'multifactorial, unpleasant emotional experience of a psychological (cognitive, emotional), social, and/or spiritual nature that may interfere with the ability to cope effectively with cancer, its physical symptoms and its treatment' [85]. Socially isolated older patients are most vulnerable to the impact of distress, which frequently goes unrecognized [86]. The NCCN guidelines endorse a simple distress 'thermometer', which consists of a single question asking the patient to characterize their level of distress on a scale of 0–10 [87]. A score of ≥4 on the distress thermometer correlates with scores on other standardized depression scales, and warrants further evaluation [88–90].

Distress is a term that encompasses a variety of psychological states including depression. Studies have demonstrated that 20–25% of older adults with cancer have unrecognized and undiagnosed depression. Depression in older adults is associated with functional decline, a need for a caregiver and caregiver stress, and increased utilization of healthcare resources [91, 92]. Screening tools include the Geriatric Depression Scale [93] and Hospital Anxiety and Depression Scale [94]. Depression in older adults can be mistaken for tumor- and treatment-related symptoms. Recent studies have identified depression as a significant prognostic factor in patients undergoing treatment for cancer [4].

Geriatric Syndromes

The term 'geriatric syndrome' is used to capture those clinical conditions in older persons that do not fit into discrete disease categories [95]. Many of the most common conditions that geriatricians treat, including delirium, falls, frailty, dizziness, and urinary incontinence, are classified as geriatric syndromes. Nevertheless, the concept of the geriatric syndrome remains poorly defined. Common themes amongst these syndromes are their prevalence amongst older frail individuals, multifactorial etiologies, and adverse impact on health outcomes. Shared risk factors for the development of geriatric syndromes include older age, baseline cognitive impairment, baseline functional impairment, and impaired mobility [95]. Koroukian et al. [96] evaluated older patients with incident breast, colon, or prostate cancer and found that greater than a third had at least one geriatric syndrome (as captured through administrative billing/database) at diagnosis. Using self-report, Mohile et al. [97] found that cancer survivors had a higher prevalence of geriatric syndromes than those without cancer. Geriatric syndromes were also found to be highly prevalent in hospitalized older cancer patients [98]. In older populations, the presence of geriatric syndromes predicts further functional decline, hospitalizations, and mortality [95, 99]. One study of colon cancer patients found that having two or more geriatric syndromes increased the likelihood of death after cancer treatment [100]. As there is limited research regarding the impact of geriatric syndromes individually or in concert on the outcomes of older patients with cancer, the CGA can help to identify geriatric syndromes that may complicate cancer care [1, 101].

Risk Stratification

Information for the CGA can be utilized to create a comprehensive review of a patient's overall health and well-being. Patients can then be risk stratified based upon deficits in the CGA, although more information is required to validate these risk-stratification schemes. Patients who have good functional and nutritional status, low level of comorbidity and strong social support are classified as 'fit' for treatment. Patients with multiple CGA deficits are considered 'frail' and would have high risk for toxicity with treatments. Those patients in-between may have modifiable risk factors and are considered 'vulnerable'. These patients are at increased risk of treatment-related toxicity as compared to 'fit' patients and should be evaluated for potential modification or dose reduction of their treatment (with escalation as tolerated) to facilitate completion of therapy with minimum toxicity.

Several recent studies have evaluated elements of the CGA to identify factors which may independently predict increased risk of chemotherapy toxicity. Hurria et al. [13] sought to identify baseline characteristics of the geriatric oncology population which would predict increased risk for grade 3, 4, or 5 toxicity. They collected pre-chemotherapy data including tumor characteristics, basic laboratory data, treatment characteristics, and CGA results on 500 patients and followed them throughout their treatment course, monitoring for toxicity events. Patients with all tumor types were included and the majority (61%) had stage IV disease. A large percentage of patients developed chemotherapy-related toxicity (39% with grade 3, 12% with grade 4, and 2% with grade 5). Nearly a third required dose reduction (31%) or had a dose delay (31%) and almost one-quarter were hospitalized during their treatment (23%). Baseline characteristics that predicted an increased risk for toxicity included age ≥72, cancer type (GI or GU malignancy), standard dosing of chemotherapy, polychemotherapy regimen, decreased hemoglobin (males <11, females <10), creatinine clearance <34, hearing impairment, one or more falls in the past 6 months, limited ability to walk one block, need for assistance with taking medications and decreased social activities. Hurria et al. [13] were able to develop a risk stratification schema by assigning a risk score for each of these factors. They demonstrated that the total risk score for a patient correlated with the incidence of treatment-related toxicity events. This tool is currently in the process of being validated in an external cohort.

A second study which developed The Chemotherapy Risk Assessment Scale for High-Age Patients (CRASH) score in over 500 patients was led by Dr. Martine Extermann [14]. In this study, patients aged ≥70 years who were starting chemotherapy completed a geriatric assessment. Toxicity of the chemotherapy regimen was adjusted using an index to estimate the average per-patient risk of chemotherapy toxicity (the MAX2 index): severe toxicity was observed in 64% of patients. The best model included IADL score, LDH level, diastolic blood pressure, and chemotherapy toxicity: risk categories: low, 7%; medium-low, 23%; medium-high, 54%, and high, 100%, respectively (p_{trend} <0.001). Predictors of non-hematologic toxicity were hemoglobin, creatinine clearance, albumin, self-rated health, Eastern Cooperative Oncology Group performance, MMSE score, MNA score, and toxicity of the chemotherapy regimen. The best predictive model included performance status, MMSE score, MNA score, and chemotherapy toxicity: risk categories: 33, 46, 67, and 93%, respectively (p_{trend} <0.001). Information from two-thirds of the patients was used to develop the risk stratification scheme, and the tool was validated in the remaining one-third of patients. This study offers oncology the first validated tool for chemotherapy toxicity in older cancer patients.

An additional study performed by Kanesvaran et al. [4] evaluated the impact of CGA domains on overall survival and developed a prognostic scoring system including these elements for use by clinicians. This study included patients of any cancer type, stage and functional status. The majority of patients had GI, GU or lung cancer and 84.7% had advanced stage malignancy. The majority of patients (66.7%) had an EGOC PS ≥2. They performed a retrospective analysis of 249 patients to determine items from the CGA which independently affected overall survival. Factors they identified included low albumin, EGOG PS ≥2, positive geriatric depression screen, advanced stage disease, malnutrition, and advanced age were. They developed a nomogram for use by clinicians to predict 1-, 2-, and 3-year overall survival for individual patients by weighting each of these independent variables [4].

Deficits in various areas of the CGA can help identify patients who may be at increased risk with treatment or may impact overall survival. Additional research is needed to identify the optimal mode of implementing the CGA and its results into daily clinical practice and to identify interventions to improve outcomes.

Are Shorter Screening Tools for Geriatric Impairment Available for Oncology Clinics?

Despite recent studies demonstrating feasibility of CGA in oncology, adoption as the standard of care has been slow due to lack of resources and the length of time to complete [20, 102–104]. A short, simple, validated screening procedure could that could identify those patients who are at risk for further morbidity or mortality would be valuable. While impaired patients could then be offered referral to more comprehensive geriatric programs for interventions, older patients who are not at risk would be spared the time-consuming CGA. A short screening tool should exclude the possibility of vulnerability with a high negative predictive value and positive results should indicate the need for a more complete geriatric evaluation [105].

Vulnerable Elders Survey-13
The Vulnerable Elders Survey-13 (VES-13) is a self-administered survey that consists of one question for age and an additional 12 items assessing self-related health, functional capacity, and physical performance [106, 107]. In the national sample of elders from the Medicare Current Beneficiary Survey (1993–1995) used to derive the VES-13, a score of ≥3 identified 32% of individuals as vulnerable [106, 107]. This identified group had over four times the risk of death or functional decline over 2 years when compared to elders scoring <3. Higher scores on the VES-13 predict increasing risk for functional decline and/or death in community-dwelling older adults [108]. In validation studies, the VES-13 was administered over the telephone or in person and the average time elders took to complete the VES-13 was less than 5 min [109].

Because of the predictive value of the VES-13 for identifying at-risk elders in the community, further work was carried out to determine whether the VES-13 was useful as a screening tool for identifying at elders who may benefit from a CGA. A population-based analysis found that a high proportion of elders with a history of cancer also scored as 'vulnerable' on the VES-13 (45.8%) and that this prevalence was statistically significantly higher than the proportion of elders without a history of cancer who scored as 'vulnerable' (39.5%, p < 0.001) [33]. In this analysis, a cancer diagnosis was associated with an increased likelihood of having a VES-13 score of ≥3 (adjusted OR 1.26, 95% CI 1.13–1.41, RR 1.14) compared with those without cancer. In another study, 50% of older patients with prostate cancer who were receiving androgen deprivation therapy were reported to have scored as 'vulnerable' on the VES-13 [54]. In these studies, it is unclear whether a personal history of cancer or other comorbidities was independently associated with the increase in factors that are related to vulnerability. In the older prostate cancer cohort on androgen deprivation therapy [54], the VES-13 had high predictive value for identifying impairment when compared to the CGA using a cut-point of ≥3.

Other studies to further clarify the testing characteristics of the VES-13 in a more heterogeneous population of cancer patients have also been conducted. Luciani et al. [110] conducted a study to establish the accuracy of the VES-13 in predicting the presence of abnormalities revealed by CGA. The population included a group of 419 patients aged ≥70 with any history of solid or hematologic malignancy. 53% of the 419 elderly patients with cancer (mean age 76.8 years) were vulnerable on VES-13; the rates of disabilities on CGA and ADL/IADL scales were 30 and 25%, respectively. The sensitivity and specificity of VES-13 were 87 and 62%, respectively, compared to CGA.

Groningen Frailty Indicator
The Groningen Frailty Indicator (GFI) is a screening instrument developed in 1991 in the community-dwelling geriatric population. It is a 15-item survey including questions focusing on mobility/physical fitness, vision/hearing, nutrition, comorbidity, cognition, and psychosocial. The score ranges from 0 to 15 and a score of 4 or higher is considered predictive of frailty, based upon consensus of a panel of geriatric experts [111]. The GFI has been shown in studies to demonstrate high internal consistency and construct validity [112]. The GFI has been shown to moderately correlate with CGA (Pearson correlation coefficient (R^2) = 0.45) [113].

A study by Aaldriks et al. [114] evaluated the predictive value of GFI in patients scheduled to undergo chemotherapy treatment. Patients of all types and stages of cancer were included in this study and initial evaluation included screening with the GFI. The authors found that the mortality rate after initiation of chemotherapy was increased for patients with higher baseline GFI scores (hazard ratio 1.80, 95% CI 1.17–2.78). The GFI has also been evaluated as a predictive tool in a cohort of geriatric patients with lung non-small cell lung cancer treated with platinum-based doublet chemotherapy. GFI score and Geriatric Depression Scale scores predicted overall outcomes [115].

G8
The G8 is a screening tool which was developed in a cohort of geriatric cancer patients. Variables are extrapolated from the MNA, which is a nutritional assessment tool developed in the 1990s specifically for the geriatric population. The MNA

has been shown to have prognostic significance for functional status, morbidity, and mortality of the elderly in a variety of settings [116]. The G8 is an 8-item questionnaire assessing domains of nutrition, mobility, cognition, polypharmacy, age and self-perceived health status. Scoring ranges from 0 (poor status) to 17 (good prognosis) and authors recommend a score of 14 as a predictor of CGA deficits (90% sensitivity and 60% specificity). This was validated in a study comparing the G8 to the VES-13 as a predictive tool for CGA deficits in geriatric cancer patients. Sensitivity of the G8 was found to be superior to the VES-13 (76.6 vs. 68.7%). However, the specificity for CGA deficits was inferior to the VES-13 (64.4 vs. 74.3%) [117].

Due to lack of consistent results and inadequate data in specific cancer types, tools should not serve as a substitute for a full CGA. Because comparisons with CGA are fraught with limitations, prospective evaluation of the utility of screening tools to predict adverse outcomes in older patients with specific cancer types and stages is necessary.

Moving Forward Utilizing CGA to Improve Outcomes of Older Cancer Patients

A few studies have demonstrated that combining geriatric and oncologic approaches can affect decision-making for treatment in patients with advanced cancer. In the ELCAPA study, a geriatrician performed an extensive CGA for older patients to start cancer treatment and proposed a geriatric intervention plan for overall patient management (e.g., social support, nutrition, psychological support, physiotherapy, memory assessment, modification of current drugs, and/or investigations) [118]. A multidisciplinary meeting was held for discussion of each patient and decisions about the cancer treatment. After the CGA, the initial cancer treatment plan was modified for 78 (20.8%) of 375 patients (95% CI 16.8–25.3), usually to decrease treatment intensity (63 (80.8%) of 78 patients). By multivariate analysis, factors independently associated with cancer treatment changes were a lower ADL score and malnutrition. In another study of 161 patients (>50% with advanced cancer), geriatric consultations impacted treatment decisions in the majority of patients; cancer treatment was changed in 79 patients (49%), including delayed therapy in 5 patients, less intensive therapy in 29 patients and, interestingly, more intensive therapy in 45 patients [119]. Patients for whom the final decision was delayed or who underwent less intensive therapy had significantly more frequent severe comorbidities (23/34, $p < 0.01$) and dependence for at least one ADL (19/34, $p < 0.01$). In a pilot study, Horgan et al. [120] demonstrated that the majority of eligible older patients were not referred for geriatric assessment, but that geriatric assessment did guide initial decision-making in those that were referred. In a study by McCorkle et al. [121], geriatric nurse practitioners conducted in-home assessments of cancer patients treated surgically, and this led to a survival advantage: a 2-year survival rate of 67% in the intervention group compared with 40% in the control group. Goodwin et al. [122] assessed the impact of nurse care management in the treatment of older women with breast cancer. Patients in the intervention arm received a geriatric assessment along plus interventions such as emotional and social support to the patient and family, help in communication of patient concerns to the treating physicians, teaching about cancer and its treatment, and referrals to other resources (e.g., support groups, home healthcare). The patients in the geriatric assessment-driven interventions group were significantly more likely to return to normal functioning than the controls.

It is likely that support from a multidisciplinary team can help develop interventions for an at-risk older adult with cancer. This team could include expertise from social work, physical therapy, occupational therapy, and nutrition. More research is now needed on how to incorporate CGA results into clinical interventions to improve outcomes.

Conclusion

The incidence of cancer increases with advanced age. The geriatric population is a heterogeneous group and a patient's chronologic age does not reflect their overall health status. Therefore, oncologists need to be adept at assessing physiologic and functional capacity in older patients. The CGA is the gold standard for evaluation of the geriatric patient. The various components of the CGA have been shown to help identify deficits missed by standard performance status and to predict outcomes including chemotherapy toxicity and survival. The combined data from the CGA can be used to stratify patients into risk categories to better predict their tolerance to treatment and risk for chemotherapy toxicity. However, the CGA is a comprehensive tool requiring significant time and training to perform. Therefore, a variety of screening tools have been developed which may be useful in the general oncology practice setting to identify patients that may benefit from further testing and intervention. Further research is still needed to evaluate whether these screening tools can predict cancer-related outcomes in older patients. Further research is also needed to help identify interventions based on CGA results that could improve outcomes of older patients with cancer.

References

1 Extermann M, Hurria A: Comprehensive Geriatric Assessment for older patients with cancer. J Clin Oncol 2007;25:1824–1831.
2 Freyer G, Geay JF, Touzet S, et al: Comprehensive Geriatric Assessment predicts tolerance to chemotherapy and survival in elderly patients with advanced ovarian carcinoma: a GINECO study. Ann Oncol 2005;16:1795–1800.
3 Pentheroudakis G, Fountzilas G, Kalofonos HP, et al: Palliative chemotherapy in elderly patients with common metastatic malignancies: A Hellenic Cooperative Oncology Group registry analysis of management, outcome and clinical benefit predictors. Crit Rev Oncol Hematol 2008;66:237–247.
4 Kanesvaran R, Li H, Koo KN, Poon D: Analysis of prognostic factors of Comprehensive Geriatric Assessment and development of a clinical scoring system in elderly Asian patients with cancer. J Clin Oncol 2011;29:3620–3627.

5 Repetto L, Fratino L, Audisio RA, et al: Comprehensive Geriatric Assessment adds information to Eastern Cooperative Oncology Group performance status in elderly cancer patients: an Italian Group for Geriatric Oncology Study. J Clin Oncol 2002; 20:494–502.
6 Katz S, Ford AB, Moskowitz RW, et al: Studies of illness in the aged. The index of ADL: a standardized measure of biological and psychosocial function. JAMA 1963;185:914–919.
7 Lawton MP, Brody EM: Assessment of older people: self-maintaining and instrumental activities of daily living. Gerontologist 1969;9:179–186.
8 Wedding U, Rohrig B, Klippstein A, Pientka L, Hoffken K: Age, severe comorbidity and functional impairment independently contribute to poor survival in cancer patients. J Cancer Res Clin Oncol 2007;133:945–950.
9 Patel KV, Peek MK, Wong R, Markides KS: Comorbidity and disability in elderly Mexican and Mexican American adults: findings from Mexico and the southwestern United States. J Aging Health 2006; 18:315–329.
10 Extermann M, Meyer J, McGinnis M, et al: A comprehensive geriatric intervention detects multiple problems in older breast cancer patients. Crit Rev Oncol Hematol 2004;49:69–75.
11 Girre V, Falcou MC, Gisselbrecht M, et al: Does a geriatric oncology consultation modify the cancer treatment plan for elderly patients? J Gerontol A Biol Sci Med Sci 2008;63:724–730.
12 Retornaz F, Monette J, Batist G, et al: Usefulness of frailty markers in the assessment of the health and functional status of older cancer patients referred for chemotherapy: a pilot study. J Gerontol A Biol Sci Med Sci 2008;63:518–522.
13 Hurria A, Togawa K, Mohile SG, et al: Predicting chemotherapy toxicity in older adults with cancer: a prospective multicenter study. J Clin Oncol 2011;29: 3457–3465.
14 Extermann M, Boler I, Reich RR, et al: Predicting the risk of chemotherapy toxicity in older patients: The Chemotherapy Risk Assessment Scale for High-Age Patients (CRASH) score. Cancer 2012; 118:3377–3386.
15 Guralnik JM, Simonsick EM, Ferrucci L, et al: A Short Physical Performance Battery assessing lower extremity function: association with self-reported disability and prediction of mortality and nursing home admission. J Gerontol 1994;49:M85–M94.
16 Rantanen T, Guralnik JM, Foley D, et al: Midlife hand grip strength as a predictor of old age disability. JAMA 1999;281:558–560.
17 Podsiadlo D, Richardson S: The timed 'up & go': a test of basic functional mobility for frail elderly persons. J Am Geriatr Soc 1991;39:142–148.
18 Guralnik JM, Ferrucci L, Pieper CF, et al: Lower extremity function and subsequent disability: consistency across studies, predictive models, and value of gait speed alone compared with the Short Physical Performance Battery. J Gerontol A Biol Sci Med Sci 2000;55:M221–M231.
19 Bylow K, Dale W, Mustian K, et al: Falls and physical performance deficits in older patients with prostate cancer undergoing androgen deprivation therapy. Urology 2008;72:422–427.
20 Hurria A, Gupta S, Zauderer M, et al: Developing a cancer-specific geriatric assessment: a feasibility study. Cancer 2005;104:1998–2005.
21 Carlson RW, Moench S, Hurria A, et al: NCCN Task Force Report: breast cancer in the older woman. J Natl Compr Canc Netw 2008;6(suppl 4):S1–S27.
22 Wildiers H, Kunkler I, Biganzoli L, et al: Management of breast cancer in elderly individuals: recommendations of the International Society of Geriatric Oncology. Lancet Oncol 2007;8:1101–1115.
23 Hurria A, Browner IS, Cohen HJ, et al: Senior adult oncology. J Natl Compr Canc Netw 2012;10:162–209.
24 Yancik R: Cancer burden in the aged: an epidemiologic and demographic overview. Cancer 1997;80: 1273–1283.
25 Extermann M: Measurement and impact of comorbidity in older cancer patients. Crit Rev Oncol Hematol 2000;35:181–200.
26 Yancik R, Havlik RJ, Wesley MN, et al: Cancer and comorbidity in older patients: a descriptive profile. Ann Epidemiol 1996;6:399–412.
27 Satariano WA, Ragland DR: The effect of comorbidity on 3-year survival of women with primary breast cancer. Ann Intern Med 1994;120:104–110.
28 Yancik R, Wesley MN, Ries LA, et al: Comorbidity and age as predictors of risk for early mortality of male and female colon carcinoma patients: a population-based study. Cancer 1998;82:2123–2134.
29 Wildes TM, Augustin KM, Sempek D, et al: Comorbidities, not age, impact outcomes in autologous stem cell transplant for relapsed non-Hodgkin lymphoma. Biology of blood and marrow transplantation. J Am Soc Blood Marrow Transplant 2008;14: 840–846.
30 Keating NL, O'Malley AJ, Freedland SJ, Smith MR: Does comorbidity influence the risk of myocardial infarction or diabetes during androgen-deprivation therapy for prostate cancer? Eur Urol 2012, E-pub ahead of print.

31 Nguyen PL, Chen MH, Beckman JA, et al: Influence of androgen deprivation therapy on all-cause mortality in men with high-risk prostate cancer and a history of congestive heart failure or myocardial infarction. Int J Radiat Oncol Biol Phys 2012;82: 1411–1416.

32 Meyerhardt JA, Catalano PJ, Haller DG, et al: Impact of diabetes mellitus on outcomes in patients with colon cancer. J Clin Oncol 2003;21:433–440.

33 Mohile SG, Xian Y, Dale W, et al: Association of a cancer diagnosis with vulnerability and frailty in older Medicare beneficiaries. J Natl Cancer Inst 2009;101:1206–1215.

34 Arias E: United States life tables, 2003. Natl Vital Stat Rep 2006;54:1–40.

35 Walters SJ, Campbell MJ, Lall R: Design and analysis of trials with quality of life as an outcome: a practical guide. J Biopharm Stat 2001;11:155–176.

36 Hamberg P, Verweij J, Seynaeve C: Cytotoxic therapy for the elderly with metastatic breast cancer: a review on safety, pharmacokinetics and efficacy. Eur J Cancer 2007;43:1514–1528.

37 Hurria A, Lichtman SM: Clinical pharmacology of cancer therapies in older adults. Br J Cancer 2008;3: 517–522.

38 Corcoran M: Polypharmacy in the older patient with cancer. Cancer Control 1997;4:419–428.

39 Sokol K, Knudsen JF, Li MM: Polypharmacy in older oncology patients and the need for an interdisciplinary approach to side-effect management. J Clin Pharm Ther 2007;32:169–175.

40 Barnett MJ, Perry PJ, Langstaff JD, Kaboli PJ: Comparison of rates of potentially inappropriate medication use according to the Zhan criteria for VA versus private sector Medicare HMOs. J Manag Care Pharm 2006;12:362–370.

41 Blalock SJ, Byrd JE, Hansen RA, et al: Factors associated with potentially inappropriate drug utilization in a sample of rural community-dwelling older adults. Am J Geriatr Pharmacother 2005;3:168–179.

42 Bregnhoj L, Thirstrup S, Kristensen MB, Bjerrum L, Sonne J: Combined intervention programme reduces inappropriate prescribing in elderly patients exposed to polypharmacy in primary care. Eur J Clin Pharmacol 2009;65:199–207.

43 Buck MD, Atreja A, Brunker CP, et al: Potentially inappropriate medication prescribing in outpatient practices: prevalence and patient characteristics based on electronic health records. Am J Geriatr Pharmacother 2009;7:84–92.

44 Flood K, Carroll MB, Le CV, Ball L, Esker DA, Carr DB: Geriatric syndromes in elderly patients admitted to an oncology-acute care for elders unit. J Clin Oncol 2006;24:2298–2303.

45 Ingram S, Seo PH, Martell RE, Clipp EC, Doyle ME, Montana GS, et al: Comprehensive assessment of the elderly cancer patient: the feasibility of self-report methodology. J Clin Oncol 2002;20:770–775.

46 Fick DM, Cooper JW, Wade WE, et al: Updating the Beers criteria for potentially inappropriate medication use in older adults: results of a US consensus panel of experts. Arch Intern Med 2003;163: 2716–2724.

47 Nahin RL, Fitzpatrick AL, Williamson JD, et al: Use of herbal medicine and other dietary supplements in community-dwelling older people: baseline data from the ginkgo evaluation of memory study. J Am Geriatr Soc 2006;54:1725–1735.

48 Gray SL, Mahoney JE, Blough DK: Medication adherence in elderly patients receiving home health services following hospital discharge. Ann Pharmacother 2001;35:539–545.

49 He SM, Yang AK, Li XT, et al: Effects of herbal products on the metabolism and transport of anti-cancer agents. Expert Opin Drug Metab Toxicol 2010;6:1195–1213.

50 Hanlon JT, Weinberger M, Samsa GP, et al: A randomized, controlled trial of a clinical pharmacist intervention to improve inappropriate prescribing in elderly outpatients with polypharmacy. Am J Med 1996;100:428–437.

51 Vinks TH, Egberts TC, de Lange TM, de Koning FH: Pharmacist-based medication review reduces potential drug-related problems in the elderly: the SMOG controlled trial. Drugs Aging 2009;26:123–133.

52 Crotty M, Rowett D, Spurling L, et al: Does the addition of a pharmacist transition coordinator improve evidence-based medication management and health outcomes in older adults moving from the hospital to a long-term care facility? Results of a randomized, controlled trial. Am J Geriatr Pharmacother 2004;2:257–264.

53 Extermann M, Aapro M: Assessment of the older cancer patient. Hematol Oncol Clin North Am 2000;14:63–77, viii–ix.

54 Mohile SG, Bylow K, Dale W, et al: A pilot study of the Vulnerable Elders Survey-13 compared with the Comprehensive Geriatric Assessment for identifying disability in older patients with prostate cancer who receive androgen ablation. Cancer 2007;109: 802–810.

55 Plassman BL, Langa KM, Fisher GG, et al: Prevalence of dementia in the United States: the aging, demographics, and memory study. Neuroepidemiology 2007;29:125–132.

56 Plassman BL, Langa KM, Fisher GG, et al: Prevalence of cognitive impairment without dementia in the United States. Ann Intern Med 2008;148:427–434.

57 Kelley BJ, Petersen RC: Alzheimer's disease and mild cognitive impairment. Neurol Clin 2007;25: 577–609.
58 Petersen RC: Mild cognitive impairment as a diagnostic entity. J Intern Med 2004;256:183–194.
59 Wolfson C, Wolfson DB, Asgharian M, et al: A reevaluation of the duration of survival after the onset of dementia. N Engl J Med 2001;344:1111–1116.
60 Dees EC, O'Reilly S, Goodman SN, et al: A prospective pharmacologic evaluation of age-related toxicity of adjuvant chemotherapy in women with breast cancer. Cancer Invest 2000;18:521–529.
61 Gupta SK, Lamont EB: Patterns of presentation, diagnosis, and treatment in older patients with colon cancer and comorbid dementia. J Am Geriatr Soc 2004;52:1681–1687.
62 Heck JE, Albert SM, Franco R, Gorin SS: Patterns of dementia diagnosis in surveillance, epidemiology, and end results breast cancer survivors who use chemotherapy. J Am Geriatr Soc 2008;56:1687–1692.
63 Gorin SS, Heck JE, Albert S, Hershman D: Treatment for breast cancer in patients with Alzheimer's disease. J Am Geriatr Soc 2005;53:1897–1904.
64 Goodwin JS, Samet JM, Hunt WC: Determinants of survival in older cancer patients. J Natl Cancer Inst 1996;88:1031–1038.
65 Hurria A, Goldfarb S, Rosen C, et al: Effect of adjuvant breast cancer chemotherapy on cognitive function from the older patient's perspective. Breast Cancer Res Treat 2006;98:343–348.
66 Chen H, Cantor A, Meyer J, et al: Can older cancer patients tolerate chemotherapy? A prospective pilot study. Cancer 2003;97:1107–1114.
67 Chodosh J, Petitti DB, Elliott M, et al: Physician recognition of cognitive impairment: evaluating the need for improvement. J Am Geriatr Soc 2004;52: 1051–1059.
68 Blessed G, Tomlinson BE, Roth M: The association between quantitative measures of dementia and of senile change in the cerebral grey matter of elderly subjects. Br J Psychiatry 1968;114:797–811.
69 Folstein MF, Folstein SE, McHugh PR: 'Mini-mental state'. A practical method for grading the cognitive state of patients for the clinician. J Psychiatr Res 1975;12:189–198.
70 Borson S, Scanlan JM, Chen P, Ganguli M: The Mini-Cog as a screen for dementia: validation in a population-based sample. J Am Geriatr Soc 2003; 51:1451–1454.
71 Pfeiffer E: A Short Portable Mental Status Questionnaire for the assessment of organic brain deficit in elderly patients. J Am Geriatr Soc 1975;23:433–441.
72 Fried LP, Kronmal RA, Newman AB, et al: Risk factors for 5-year mortality in older adults: the Cardiovascular Health Study. JAMA 1998;279:585–592.
73 Diehr P, Bild DE, Harris TB, et al: Body mass index and mortality in nonsmoking older adults: the Cardiovascular Health Study. Am J Public Health 1998; 88:623–629.
74 Dewys WD, Begg C, Lavin PT, et al: Prognostic effect of weight loss prior to chemotherapy in cancer patients. Eastern Cooperative Oncology Group. Am J Med 1980;69:491–497.
75 Vellas B, Guigoz Y, Garry PJ, et al: The Mini Nutritional Assessment (MNA) and its use in grading the nutritional state of elderly patients. Nutrition 1999; 15:116–122.
76 Seeman TE, Berkman LF, Kohout F, Lacroix A, Glynn R, Blazer D: Intercommunity variations in the association between social ties and mortality in the elderly. A comparative analysis of three communities. Ann Epidemiol 1993;3:325–335.
77 Kroenke CH, Kubzansky LD, Schernhammer ES, et al: Social networks, social support, and survival after breast cancer diagnosis. J Clin Oncol 2006;24: 1105–1111.
78 Osborne C, Ostir GV, Du X, et al: The influence of marital status on the stage at diagnosis, treatment, and survival of older women with breast cancer. Breast Cancer Res Treat 2005;93:41–47.
79 Bernabei R, Venturiero V, Tarsitani P, Gambassi G: The Comprehensive Geriatric Assessment: when, where, how. Crit Rev Oncol Hematol 2000;33:45–56.
80 Bried EM, Scheffler RM: The financial stages of cancer in the elderly. Oncology (Williston Park) 1992;6(suppl):153–160.
81 Warren JL, Brown ML, Fay MP, et al: Costs of treatment for elderly women with early-stage breast cancer in fee-for-service settings. J Clin Oncol 2002;20: 307–316.
82 Penberthy L, Retchin SM, McDonald MK, et al: Predictors of Medicare costs in elderly beneficiaries with breast, colorectal, lung, or prostate cancer. Health Care Manag Sci 1999;2:149–160.
83 Mandelblatt JS, Edge SB, Meropol NJ, et al: Predictors of long-term outcomes in older breast cancer survivors: perceptions versus patterns of care. J Clin Oncol 2003;21:855–863.
84 Vinokur AD, Threatt BA, Vinokur-Kaplan D, Satariano WA: The process of recovery from breast cancer for younger and older patients. Changes during the first year. Cancer 1990;65:1242–1254.
85 Holland JC, Bultz BD: The NCCN guideline for distress management: a case for making distress the sixth vital sign. J Natl Compr Canc Netw 2007;5:3–7.
86 Sollner W, DeVries A, Steixner E, et al: How successful are oncologists in identifying patient distress, perceived social support, and need for psychosocial counselling? Br J Cancer 2001;84:179–185.

87 Hoffman BM, Zevon MA, D'Arrigo MC, Cecchini TB: Screening for distress in cancer patients: the NCCN rapid-screening measure. Psychooncology 2004;13:792–799.

88 Roth AJ, Kornblith AB, Batel-Copel L, Peabody E, Scher HI, Holland JC: Rapid screening for psychologic distress in men with prostate carcinoma: a pilot study. Cancer 1998;82:1904–1908.

89 Ransom S, Jacobsen PB, Booth-Jones M: Validation of the distress thermometer with bone marrow transplant patients. Psychooncology 2006;15:604–612.

90 Jacobsen PB, Donovan KA, Trask PC, et al: Screening for psychologic distress in ambulatory cancer patients. Cancer 2005;103:1494–1502.

91 Penninx BW, Guralnik JM, Ferrucci L, Simonsick EM, Deeg DJ, Wallace RB: Depressive symptoms and physical decline in community-dwelling older persons. JAMA 1998;279:1720–1726.

92 Langa KM, Valenstein MA, Fendrick AM, Kabeto MU, Vijan S: Extent and cost of informal caregiving for older Americans with symptoms of depression. Am J Psychiatry 2004;161:857–863.

93 Yesavage JA, Brink TL, Rose TL, et al: Development and validation of a geriatric depression screening scale: a preliminary report. J Psychiatr Res 1982;17:37–49.

94 Zigmond AS, Snaith RP: The hospital anxiety and depression scale. Acta Psychiatr Scand 1983;67:361–370.

95 Inouye SK, Studenski S, Tinetti ME, Kuchel GA: Geriatric syndromes: clinical, research, and policy implications of a core geriatric concept. J Am Geriatr Soc 2007;55:780–791.

96 Koroukian SM, Murray P, Madigan E: Comorbidity, disability, and geriatric syndromes in elderly cancer patients receiving home health care. J Clin Oncol 2006;24:2304–2310.

97 Mohile SG, Fan L, Reeve E, et al: Association of cancer with geriatric syndromes in older Medicare beneficiaries. J Clin Oncol 2011;29:1458–1464.

98 Flood KL, Carroll MB, Le CV, Ball L, Esker DA, Carr DB: Geriatric syndromes in elderly patients admitted to an oncology – acute care for elders unit. J Clin Oncol 2006;24:2298–2303.

99 Anpalahan M, Gibson SJ: Geriatric syndromes as predictors of adverse outcomes of hospitalization. Intern Med J 2008;38:16–23.

100 Koroukian SM, Xu F, Bakaki PM, et al: Comorbidities, functional limitations, and geriatric syndromes in relation to treatment and survival patterns among elders with colorectal cancer. J Gerontol A Biol Sci Med Sci 2010;65:322–329.

101 Wedding U, Hoffken K: Care of breast cancer in the elderly woman – what does Comprehensive Geriatric Assessment (CGA) help? Support Care Cancer 2003;11:769–774.

102 Ingram SS, Seo PH, Martell RE, et al: Comprehensive assessment of the elderly cancer patient: the feasibility of self-report methodology. J Clin Oncol 2002;20:770–775.

103 Hurria A, Lachs MS, Cohen HJ, et al: Geriatric assessment for oncologists: rationale and future directions. Crit Rev Oncol Hematol 2006;59:211–217.

104 Hurria A: Incorporation of geriatric principles in oncology clinical trials. J Clin Oncol 2007;25:5350–5351.

105 Molina-Garrido MJ, Guillen-Ponce C: Overvaluation of the Vulnerable Elders Survey-13 as a screening tool for vulnerability. J Clin Oncol 2011;29:3201–3203.

106 Saliba D, Orlando M, Wenger NS, et al: Identifying a short functional disability screen for older persons. J Gerontol A Biol Sci Med Sci 2000;55:M750–M756.

107 Saliba D, Elliott M, Rubenstein LZ, et al: The Vulnerable Elders Survey: a tool for identifying vulnerable older people in the community. J Am Geriatr Soc 2001;49:1691–1699.

108 Min LC, Elliott MN, Wenger NS, Saliba D: Higher Vulnerable Elders Survey scores predict death and functional decline in vulnerable older people. J Am Geriatr Soc 2006;54:507–511.

109 Wenger NS, Solomon DH, Roth CP, et al: The quality of medical care provided to vulnerable community-dwelling older patients. Ann Intern Med 2003;139:740–747.

110 Luciani A, Ascione G, Bertuzzi C, et al: Detecting disabilities in older patients with cancer: comparison between Comprehensive Geriatric Assessment and Vulnerable Elders Survey-13. J Clin Oncol 2010;28:2046–2050.

111 Steverink N, Slaets JP, Schuurmans H, van Lis M: Measuring frailty: developing and testing the GFI (Groningen Frailty Indicator). Gerontologist 2001;41:236.

112 Metzelthin SF, Daniels R, van Rossum E, de Witte L, van den Heuvel WJ, Kempen GI: The psychometric properties of three self-report screening instruments for identifying frail older people in the community. BMC Public Health 2010;10:176.

113 Schrijvers D, Baitar A, De Vos M, et al: Evaluation of the Groningen Frailty Index (GFI) as a screening tool in elderly patients: an interim analysis. 2009. http://www.cancer.gov/clinicaltrials/search/view/print?cdrid=658351&version=HealthProfessional.

114 Aaldriks AA, Maartense E, le Cessie S, et al: Predictive value of geriatric assessment for patients older than 70 years, treated with chemotherapy. Crit Rev Oncol Hematol 2011;79:205–212.

115 Biesma B, Wymenga AN, Vincent A, et al: Quality of life, geriatric assessment and survival in elderly patients with non-small-cell lung cancer treated with carboplatin-gemcitabine or carboplatin-paclitaxel: NVALT-3 a phase III study. Ann Oncol 2011; 22:1520–1527.

116 Bauer JM, Kaiser MJ, Anthony P, et al: The Mini-Nutritional Assessment – its history, today's practice, and future perspectives. Nutr Clin Pract 2008; 23:388–396.

117 Soubeyran P, Bellera C, Goyard J, et al: Validation of the G8 screening tool in geriatric oncology: the ONCODAGE project. J Clin Oncol 2011;29(suppl): abstr 9001.

118 Caillet P, Canoui-Poitrine F, Vouriot J, et al: Comprehensive Geriatric Assessment in the decision-making process in elderly patients with cancer: ELCAPA study. J Clin Oncol 2011;29:3636–3642.

119 Chaibi P, Magne N, Breton S, et al: Influence of geriatric consultation with Comprehensive Geriatric Assessment on final therapeutic decision in elderly cancer patients. Crit Rev Oncol Hematol 2011;79: 302–307.

120 Horgan AM, Leighl NB, Coate L, et al: Impact and feasibility of a comprehensive geriatric assessment in the oncology setting: a pilot study. Am J Clin Oncol 2012;35:322–328.

121 McCorkle R, Strumpf NE, Nuamah IF, et al: A specialized home care intervention improves survival among older post-surgical cancer patients. J Am Geriatr Soc 2000;48:1707–1713.

122 Goodwin JS, Satish S, Anderson ET, et al: Effect of nurse case management on the treatment of older women with breast cancer. J Am Geriatr Soc 2003; 51:1252–1259.

Supriya G. Mohile, MD, MS
School of Medicine and Dentistry
University of Rochester Medical Center
601 Elmwood Avenue, Box 704, Rochester, NY 14642 (USA)
E-Mail supriya_mohile@urmc.rochester.edu

Pharmacology of Aging and Cancer: How Useful Are Pharmacokinetic Tests?

Stuart M. Lichtman

Memorial Sloan-Kettering Cancer Center, Commack, N.Y. and Weill Cornell Medical College, New York, N.Y., USA

Abstract

The elderly comprise the majority of patients with cancer and are the recipients of the greatest amount of chemotherapy. Unfortunately, there is a lack of data to make evidence-based decisions with regard to chemotherapy. This is due to the minimal participation of older patients in clinical trials and that trials have not systematically evaluated chemotherapy. This chapter reviews the available information with regard to chemotherapy and aging. Due to the lack of prospective data, the conclusions and recommendations made are a consensus of the available information. Extrapolation of data from younger to older patients is necessary, particularly to those patients older than 80 years, for which data is almost entirely lacking. The classes of drugs reviewed include alkylators, antimetabolites, platinum compounds, anthracyclines, taxanes, purine analogues, antimicrotubule agents, camptothecins, and epipodophyllotoxins. Clinical trials need to incorporate an analysis of chemotherapy in terms of the pharmacokinetic and pharmacodynamic effects of aging. In addition, data already accumulated need to be re-analyzed by age to aid in the management of the older cancer patient.

Copyright © 2013 S. Karger AG, Basel

Background

The study of the pharmacokinetics of chemotherapy in older patients has truly been lacking. This has been primarily due to a general exclusion of the elderly from clinical trials. This has been a persistent underrepresentation of older patients from trials which has resulted in the approval of drugs by the Food and Drug Administration [1, 2]. This has led to a paucity of data available to the clinician to make rational treatment decisions. Most, but certainly not all, of the available literature is based on retrospective, subset analyses in which older patients represent a small proportion of the total population. Patients reported generally do not have significant comorbidity and may not be truly representation of the average patient seen in practice. There is very little prospective pharmacokinetic data. Many papers focus on toxicity, which reflects pharmacodynamic changes in the older patient. In addition to age, there have been a number of publications regarding end-organ dysfunction. While this is not specifically for the elderly, the data can be utilized for this purpose as older patients have a higher incidence of comorbidity. Because of the overall lack of data, particularly for patients over the age of 80 years, the clinician will continue to have the task of extrapolating data to fit the individual patient. Clinical judgment will always be important. Modification of toxicity and appropriateness of dosing will also be affected by the use of hematopoietic growth factors and change in the schedule of drug administration [3]. The assessment of renal function is extraordinarily important in dosing chemotherapy. There is controversy which formula is the most accurate in the elderly. It is clear that serum creatinine should not be the sole determinant of renal function in the elderly or in patients with cachexia [4–7].

Should We Study Pharmacokinetics and Pharmacodynamics in Older Patients?

Is there a need to study pharmacokinetics in older patients? If we say that it is not necessary, then we are saying that our current clinical trials structure is adequate for older patients. It is definitely not, as indicated by the underrepresentation of these patients in trials. In terms of drug trials, the pharmacokinetics of current chemotherapy has been primarily studied in the 'typical' patients. That is, those patients without significant comorbidity and good performance and functional status. End-organ dysfunction studies have been performed on many drugs such as irinotecan, paclitaxel, gemcitabine, pemetrexed [8–11]. To date, there are few studies which have shown a difference between the 'typical' patients and elderly. Few age-related changes have been reported. Pharmacokinetic differences, when present, have not been clinically relevant. In addition, there are virtually no studies which look at changes in pharmacokinetics over multiple cycles. Heterogeneity makes studies in the elderly difficult and results in too much variability to be clinically applicable. Some differences in clinical toxicity have often been a result of drug scheduling, not age [12]. An example, whether 5-fluorouracil (5-FU) toxicity differs if administered weekly, as a bolus monthly or as infusion.

One rationale in the past to do pharmacokinetics studies was the avoidance of toxicity. Hematologic toxicity has been minimized due to hematopoietic growth factors. Dose-limiting toxicity is often due to non-hematologic toxicities which are not related to significant differences in pharmacokinetics, i.e. neuropathy from oxaliplatin.

One main issue is to determine which subset of elderly patients should be chosen to do pharmacokinetic studies. Are they the healthy, vulnerable, frail, anemic, hypoalbuminemic, those dependent in activities of daily living (ADL) or instrumental ADL (IADL) and multiple comorbidities? Many older patients have had previous chemotherapy and radiation for treatment of other cancers. In addition, comorbidity may causes further change in organ function and change the patients' sensitivity to toxicity, i.e., diabetes-neuropathy, atherosclerotic heart disease-cardiomyopathy. We should be studying pharmacokinetic tests in these different elderly populations. The factors to be studied should also include oral therapy, compliance, biologic therapy, and drug interactions. The other factors which should be included in data acquisition include longitudinal effects of treatment, changes in cognition, changes in function with treatment, dependency, chronic toxicities, scheduling differences which can effect toxicity, and correlation of toxicity and function. The inclusion of pharmacogenomics is also critical [13]. In evaluating toxicity, one question which needs to be answered is: Are our toxicity scales adequate for older patients? Do they capture enough information, particularly function, such as the effect of neuropathy.

Therefore, pharmacokinetics should be studied but the trials need to be novel and include these aforementioned factors. Regulatory agencies should require the inclusion of older patients before drugs can be approved.

The pharmacokinetics of common chemotherapeutic agents are discussed with emphasis on older patients.

Alkylating Agents

Alkylating agents have been the foundation of therapy for decades, particularly for breast cancer and hematologic malignancies. Their main dose-limiting toxicity is the hematologic. The large interindividual variability in bone marrow reserves is well known among older patients depending on comorbidity. Metabolism represents the main route of elimination for most compounds. Hepatic enzymatic processes are often involved [14]. Cytotoxic effects correspond to metabolites rather to parent compounds.

Melphalan
Melphalan is administered to elderly patients for treatment of multiple myeloma. Drug excreted unchanged in the urine represents about one third of the administered dose [15]. Positive correlation has been observed between melphalan area under the curve (AUC) and the degree of renal insufficiency [16, 17]. However, renal insufficiency did lead to a limited decrease in melphalan clearance compared to the interindividual variations in systemic clearance [18, 19].

High-dose chemotherapy is being increasingly utilized for the treatment of multiple myeloma in older patients [20–23]. Doses up to 200 mg/m^2 by intravenous infusion have become a standard. Higher toxicity, mainly myelosuppression, has been observed in patients over the age of 70 years [23, 24]. There is no recommendation of melphalan dosing based on renal function, but there is a consensus that reduction of the melphalan dose should be considered in patients with a glomerular filtration rate (GFR) of <30 ml/min. There are a number of treatment options available for elderly patients with multiple myeloma ineligible for high-dose chemotherapy [25, 26]. The treatment of myeloma has evolved and there other treatments not involving traditional alkylating agents [27].

Cyclophosphamide
Metabolism of cyclophosphamide to active metabolites is initiated by cytochrome P450 (subfamily 3A and 2B) mainly in the liver. An accumulation of toxic alkylating metabolites is expected in renal insufficiency justifying a dose reduction of 20–30% depending on the degree of the renal insufficiency [28]. Cyclophosphamide is administered in combination with methotrexate and 5-FU (CMF) for treatment of breast cancer. A prospective study in patients over 70 years of age concluded that the dose of CMF in patients over 70 years should not exceed 75% of the standard dose [29]. The combination cyclophosphamide/doxorubicin for the treatment for breast cancer was evaluated [30]. There was moderate evidence of an age-related decrease in the nadir absolute neutrophil count. Pharmacokinetic analyses did not demonstrate age-related differences in the either cyclophosphamide or doxorubicin plasma exposure, but only the pharmacokinetics of the parent drug (unchanged cyclophosphamide) was explored. Overall, regarding the modest effect of age on toxicity, the authors concluded that healthy older patients should not be denied adjuvant chemotherapy. The available evidence indicates that dose modification is not required due to age alone.

Bendamustine
Bendamustine is a novel chemotherapeutic agent comprised of a bifunctional mechlorethamine alkylating group, a purine-like benzimidazole ring, and a butyric acid side chain. The drug has been shown to be a potent cytotoxic agent, with in vitro studies demonstrating extensive and durable DNA damage. It has activity in various hematologic malignancies [31–34]. In a pharmacokinetic trial, bendamustine was administered as a 60-min 120 mg/m^2 intravenous infusion on days 1 and 2 of six 21-day cycles [35]. Pharmacokinetic models were developed with covariate assessment. Following a single dose of bendamustine HCl, concentrations declined in a triphasic manner, with rapid distribution, intermediate, and slow terminal phases. The intermediate $t_{1/2}$ (40 min) was considered the pharmacologically relevant (β elimination) $t_{1/2}$ since the initial phases accounted for 99% of the AUC. Age, sex, mild/moderate renal, or mild liver impairment did not alter pharmacokinetics.

Fluoropyrimidines
Fluoropyrimidines are one of the most widely used groups of agents in the medical treatment of solid malignancies. There are marked intraindividual variations in plasma levels of the parent drug and metabolites, and that toxicities can vary widely among individuals [36]. In the elderly, these drugs are commonly reduced in dosage often arbitrarily [37].

Studies Suggesting an Effect of Age on Toxicity

Stein et al. [38] reported increased toxicity with age in a phase III trial of the Gastrointestinal Study Group treatment of metastatic colorectal cancer. This was based on a logistic regression analysis using age, gender, treatment, performance status, and length of therapy. These conclusions are also supported by data derived from a meta-analysis of six randomized trials of patients with colorectal carcinoma with a total of 1,219 patients comparing infusional 5-FU with bolus 5-FU [39]. Older patients and those with poorer performance status had significantly higher risks of diarrhea, mucositis, nausea and vomiting, and older female patients having the highest incidence of this toxicity. Grade 3 or greater hematologic toxicity was sevenfold more common with bolus 5-FU (31 vs. 4%, p < 0.0001) [39].

Studies Suggesting That Age Is Not Determinant of Toxicity

An overview of seven phase III trials involving 5-FU with either leucovorin or levamisole showed that no interaction between age and outcome could be identified. Age greater than 70 years correlated with the occurrence of treatment-related leukopenia with borderline significance [40]. In an attempt to minimize the bias of patient selection for a protocol study, Delea et al. [41] retrospectively examined a 5% sample of Medicare patients who had undergone colorectal surgery. There was no difference in the incidence of hospitalization but drug dosage and comorbid conditions were not identified. In a retrospective analysis of clinical trials testing FOLFOX 4 (5-FU, leucovorin, oxaliplatin), older age was not associated with an increased overall incidence of grade ≥3 toxicity or 60-day mortality except that there was a higher incidence of grade 3 neutropenia and thrombocytopenia. The benefit of FOLFOX4 did not differ by age [42]. In an Intergroup study with adjuvant 5-FU for high-risk stage II and stage III colon cancer, the secondary analysis of this trial demonstrated that the elderly are as likely to tolerate the benefit from adjuvant chemotherapy as are younger patients [43]. In an evaluation of the Surveillance Epidemiology and End Results Medicare-linked database for resected stage III colorectal cancer, adjuvant 5-FU was well tolerated even among the very old patients without a major comorbidity [44]. A retrospective analysis of European trials has shown equivalent benefit and toxicity in 'fit' elderly patients who benefit to the same extent as younger patients [45].

Capecitabine

Studies have compared capecitabine with 5-FU in patients with a median age over 60 years [46–51]. From this literature it appears that capecitabine at the recommended dosage of 1,250 mg/m^2 twice daily for days 1–14 every 21 days is better tolerated than 5-FU administered as per Mayo schedule 425 mg/m^2 days 1–5 every 28 days. Hand-foot syndrome is more common with the capecitabine therapy and myelosuppression more common in the 5-FU therapy. Feliu et al. [52] studied prospectively 51 patients with advanced colorectal cancer who were older than 70 years of age with doses adjusted based on creatinine clearance (CrCl). Only 12% of patients experienced grade 3 or 4 treatment-related adverse events, such as diarrhea, hand-foot syndrome and thrombocytopenia. No treatment-related deaths were reported. The median dose intensity was 88% of that predicted. Sharma et al. [53] studied the effect of fixed-dose oral capecitabine 2,000 mg twice daily on days 1–14 every 3 weeks in patients with advanced colorectal cancer with a median age of 72 years. Grade 2 and 3 treatment-related toxicities were diarrhea 34%, fatigue 27%, stomatitis 15%, and hand-foot syndrome 22%. The median overall survival was 11.2 months and the response rate was 28%. The patients with the higher pretreatment levels of serum folate experienced the greater treatment toxicities over the entire treatment period (p = 0.04). The toxicities reported could be just a consequence of impaired renal function that occurs with aging. In a prospective evaluation, Cassidy et al. [54] have found that patients with moderate renal impairment at baseline (estimated CrCl 30–50 ml/min) experienced a higher incidence of grade 3 or 4 toxicities. Therefore, the authors recommended a lower starting dose in patients with moderate renal impairment at baseline (calculated CrCl 30–50 ml/min) and a contraindication in patients with severely impaired CrCl at baseline (<30 ml/min). For patients with normal or mildly impaired renal function at baseline, the standard starting dose is well tolerated. In efforts to further improve the therapeutic index, studies have been performed which alter the schedule to 7 days on and 7 days off. This schedule may be preferable in older patients in terms of toxicity and compliance [55–57].

Data has been published giving conflicting results as to whether fluoropyrimidines are more toxic in elderly patients. A main determinant of this difference is the schedule utilized. It is clear that the weekly 5-FU regimen is better tolerated than the monthly regimen [43]. Infusional therapy likely has a more favorable toxicity profile [45]. Intravenous fluoropyrimidines should be given by a weekly schedule or by the published infusional regimens. Recent data suggest no reason to dose reduce fluoropyrimidines unless there is severe renal dysfunction, poor performance status, prior radiation therapy, or comorbidity. The dose of capecitabine should be adjusted to CrCl and a starting dose of no greater than 1,000 mg/m² twice daily be strongly considered. The interaction with coumadin needs to be emphasized in older patients [58].

Platinum Compounds

Oxaliplatin
The kidneys eliminate approximately 30–50% of the drug. Clearance of total and free platinum is decreased in patients with renal impairment. However, in studies of patients with mild to moderate renal impairment (GFR >20 ml/min), no increased toxicity was seen [59, 60]. Clearance of ultrafilterable platinum after administration of oxaliplatin is not influenced by impairment of hepatic function, sex or age [61].

Principal dose-limiting toxicities are peripheral neuropathy and bone marrow suppression. Few studies have been performed specifically in the elderly population. The retrospective meta-analysis of 3,742 patients (614 ≥70 years) performed by Goldberg et al. [42] of patients receiving FOLFOX was mentioned previously. A retrospective review of 44 patients (median age 78) concluded that treatment in this population was feasible with manageable toxicity [62]. The combination of oxaliplatin/capecitabine has been studied in patients over 70 years of age. No relationship was seen between response and patient age, ECOG performance status, or the ability to perform ADL or IADL [63, 64]. The rate of neurotoxicity secondary to oxaliplatin-based chemotherapy has not been shown to be any greater in the elderly than in younger patients; a bifractionated protocol was developed in an attempt to minimize this side effect. Grade 3 sensory neuropathy occurred in 6% of patients. ADL and IADL scores did not change significantly during treatment [65]. Other trials with oxaliplatin combinations in patients over 70 years of age showed acceptable toxicity and efficacy [66–68]. Future studies need to perform prospective evaluations of neuropathy and aging needs to be performed with an emphasis on the possibility of functional impairment and long-term toxicity.

Cisplatin

Cisplatin has triphasic elimination and shows half-life of the initial phase is 20–30 min, second-phase half-life is 48–67 min, with a terminal half-life of 24 h. Cisplatin pharmacokinetics is dependent on normal renal function due to the contribution of renal elimination for cisplatin [69]. However, the non-reversible plasma protein binding of cisplatin should be also considered as an elimination process since only the unbound plasma cisplatin concentrations represent the active fraction. Plasma protein binding of cisplatin is larger than that of other platinum compounds (e.g. carboplatin). However, renal function should be considered as the major pharmacodynamic parameter since renal insufficiency represents the major toxicity together with magnesium wasting, nausea and vomiting, peripheral neuropathy, auditory impairment, and myelosuppression. Severe nausea and vomiting has been markedly reduced as a significant toxicity by the premedication of patients with a serotonin receptor type-3 antagonist. Intravenous hydration has reduced acute nephrotoxicity to 5% but intensive hydration regimens may be difficult in older patients [70]. Dose modification based on age alone is not required. It needs to be emphasized that patients receiving cisplatin in clinical trials are a highly selected group with minimal comorbidity. Calculation of renal function is critical using one of the available formulae, but should be used with caution [4, 6, 71].

Carboplatin

Carboplatin, compared with cisplatin, has a similar mechanism of action with antineoplastic activity against cervical, lung, and ovarian cancers. Carboplatin is completely eliminated through the kidneys. The Cockcroft-Gault, Calvert, and Chatelut formulae allow for accurate and safe dosing, taking into account renal function changes with age and a targeted AUC [72–74]. Carboplatin exhibits biphasic elimination with an initial half-life of 1.1–2 h, and final half-life of 2.6–5.9 h with CrCl >60 ml/min. Because of the low incidence of non-hematologic toxicity, it can replace cisplatin in the palliative setting, particularly in older patients. Obesity, which is more common in the elderly, may affect the calculation of renal function [7, 75, 76].

Anthracyclines

Anthracyclines are part of regimens for the treatment of many malignancies encountered in the elderly [77–80]. Toxicity that is observed more frequently is a form of cardiomyopathy that manifests itself during the therapy with doxorubicin in the greatest part of the cases [81], and it has been reported that the incidence of congestive heart failure following treatment with anthracyclines increases progressively with age after 70 years [82]. This may explain why many elderly patients are either excluded from chemotherapy treatment or receive less aggressive chemotherapy. Dose modification of the adjuvant chemotherapy regimen due to obesity is not necessary [83]. For anthracyclines, some studies suggest that the drug's peak concentration correlates with efficacy when toxicity is most likely a function of both peak and exposure [84–89]. The limited sampling strategies developed for several anthracyclines would facilitate the implementation of pharmacokinetic studies [90–93]. The best example is the case of epirubicin. The studies described a triexponential model for epirubicin behavior. In one study, variability in clearance could be attributed to gender and also to age in women [94]. If severe renal impairment leads to a decrease in epirubicin clearance, no dose reduction guidelines have been proposed. The pharmacokinetic profile of epirubicin is modified in case of hepatic impairment [95, 96]. Dosing modifications based on aspartate aminotransferase levels have been proposed [97–99].

Liposomal Anthracyclines

Liposomal formulation completely alters the pharmacokinetics, pharmacodynamics and toxicity profile of these agents. Palmar-plantar erythrodysesthesia syndrome is seen more frequently with these drugs; conversely, mucositis, alopecia, and cardiac toxicity are markedly diminished compared with non-liposomal formulations [100]. The reduced toxicity of this class of drugs may be particularly beneficial in older patients with anthracycline-sensitive diseases [101–105].

Antimicrotubule Agents (Spindle Poisons) in Elderly Cancer Patients

Vinca Alkaloids

Vincristine is excreted primarily by the liver and requires dose reduction, or even avoidance, in liver failure [106–108]. There are no data for dose modification based on age alone.

Vinorelbine is a semisynthetic vinca alkaloid and causes less neurotoxicity than the older compounds in this group. It is highly bound to human platelets (78%) [109] and thrombocytopenia seems to correlate with increased hematologic toxicity, probably due to an increased unbound fraction, although high inter- and intraindividual variability in AUC (20–65%) can be present [110]. Vinorelbine undergoes substantial hepatic elimination but dose modification might only be necessary in patients with severe liver dysfunction, when the liver volume has been replaced by tumor by more than 75% [111]. There are conflicting data on the effect of age on pharmacokinetics of intravenous vinorelbine [112–114]. In the largest study, CrCl and hepatic clearance were independent factors of vinorelbine clearance while age was not [114]. Several studies in breast and lung cancer and non-Hodgkin's lymphoma show that full-dose vinorelbine (e.g. 25–30 mg/m^2 weekly with rest points) has a very favorable tolerance profile [112, 115–117], and improved quality of life has been demonstrated in a large phase III trial in NSCLC in the elderly (median age 74 years) [118]. Although there are conflicting data on the impact of age on vinorelbine exposure, several trials show that vinorelbine is generally well tolerated in elderly cancer patients. There is no evidence that dose modification is required on the basis of age.

Taxanes: Paclitaxel and Docetaxel

Paclitaxel
The majority of paclitaxel is protein bound (97%) and it is extensively metabolized in the liver by the cytochrome P450 system and is excreted in bile, more specifically by the cytochrome P450 isozymes CYP2C8 and CYP3A. Awareness of drug interactions is needed when given concomitantly with drugs metabolized by the same pathways, e.g. ketoconazole [119]. It is preferable not to use paclitaxel in liver dysfunction because of significantly increased AUC and toxicity (mostly neutropenia) [10, 106], but if it is necessary, the dose should be greatly reduced. A CALGB trial shows a modest but significant decrease in clearance of total paclitaxel with increasing age [120]. This decrease seems partly induced by decreased clearance of the formulation vehicle Cremophor EL [121]. Moreover, unbound paclitaxel might be a better predictor of clinically relevant exposure than total paclitaxel. Many studies have shown the feasibility and efficacy of administering paclitaxel in elderly patients with various cancer types. Both weekly and 3-weekly regimens have been studied. The every 3-week regimen can be used in fit elderly patients such as those with ovarian and bladder cancer [122]. There is a preference for weekly administration in some patients, particularly breast cancer, as this causes less hematological toxicity without loss of efficacy [123–125], possibly as a result of the more effective antiangiogenic activity in this fractionated regimen [126].

There are somewhat conflicting data on the impact of age on paclitaxel clearance. Moreover, the importance of unbound versus total paclitaxel clearance is not fully determined. However, several trials indicate the feasibility of both every 3-week weekly paclitaxel in elderly patients. There is no basis for a dose reduction based on age alone for any standard dose or schedule. Neurotoxicity has emerged as a significant toxicity and seems to be more significant in older patients [127, 128].

Docetaxel

The majority of docetaxel is protein bound (94%), and it is extensively metabolized in the liver by the cytochrome P450 system (CYP3A4) and excreted in bile, resulting in increased toxicity when administered to patients with impaired liver function [10]. There is a large interpatient variability in exposure (AUC) and drug clearance. Hepatic CYP3A4 is by far the strongest predictor of total docetaxel clearance, and together with α_1-acid glycoprotein (AAG) accounts for 72% of the interpatient variation in clearance [129]. In serum, docetaxel is extensively bound to albumin, lipoproteins and AAG; indeed, the latter is the main determinant of docetaxel serum binding variability. There have been attempts in elderly patients to predict variation in AUC of docetaxel through correlations with plasma (AAG) or urinary cortisol ratio [130]. Many studies have investigated the efficacy and toxicity of docetaxel in relation to age, mainly in breast cancer [131–133] lung and prostate cancer [134]. In a specific phase I trial in elderly cancer patients treated with docetaxel every 3 weeks, maximal tolerated dose was not reached at 80 mg/m^2, and accrual was continued. On the other hand, another phase I trial in elderly breast cancer patients was stopped after 4 patients at the first level of 75 mg/m^2 every 3 weeks because of excessive toxicity. The Japanese population might be more vulnerable due to ethnic differences in metabolism; the MTD in a phase I trial was 30 mg/m^2/week. As with paclitaxel, weekly dose docetaxel regimens have being investigated, and seem to decrease toxicity without loss of efficacy except maybe in prostate cancer where 3-weekly might be slightly more effective than weekly docetaxel [134]. Neutropenia was limited with weekly regimens, but fatigue was often invalidating. Various dosages (e.g. 20–35 mg/m^2 weekly or 60–100 mg/m^2 every 3 weeks) and regimens (rest weeks at various time points) have been used.

There is no significant data to support dose modification based on age alone. Docetaxel pharmacokinetics is at most only minimally influenced by age. Any age-related changes are minimal compared to interpatient variability in metabolism. However, elderly patients are somewhat more vulnerable to side effects, but also here, interpatient variability is larger than age-related variability. Improvement in predicting unbound docetaxel clearance and toxicity by pharmacogenomic-based treatment optimization will hopefully improve correct dosing for the (elderly) cancer patients. In principal, standard regimens of docetaxel can be used, e.g. 30–36 mg/m^2 weekly with a rest week at regular time points, or 75 mg/m^2 3 times weekly. The choice between weekly and 3-weekly can depend on the setting (e.g. in prostate cancer, 3-weekly at 75 mg/m^2 is the standard) and on potential side effects.

Purine Analogues

Fludarabine
The elimination half-life of this drug ranges from 6.9 to 12.4 h. The total body clearance of this agent is related to both the serum creatinine and the CrCl. After initial dephosphorylation, the subsequent metabolite, 2-fluoro-araA, is eliminated primarily be renal excretion, with approximately 60% of the administered dose excreted in the urine within 24 h after administration [135]. Dose modifications based on varying degrees of renal dysfunction have been proposed [136]. The most significant toxicities with fludarabine are related to the therapy-related myelosuppression from this agent, as well as the impact on cellular immune function. The severity of fludarabine-related neutropenia is related not only to the total body clearance of this agent, but also to AUC and half-life β. No association was found between age and the incidence of either hematologic toxicity or infection during the first cycle of fludarabine therapy. However, patients with an estimated CrCl of <80 ml/min had an increased risk of toxicity during their treatment course [137]. Fludarabine may be used efficaciously and safely in an older patient population. Response rates tend to be lower in these older patients as compared to a younger cohort. Dose reductions are recommended in the setting of reduced CrCl, in an effort to limit treatment-related toxicities.

Cytarabine
Cytarabine is rapidly metabolized in the liver to inactive metabolites and 90–96% is excreted in the urine [138]. Due to increased neurotoxicity in patients with renal insufficiency, dose adjustments are required for high-dose therapy.

Gemcitabine
Pharmacokinetic data indicate that small age- and sex-related differences exist. These differences corresponded to differences in mean half-life for men at 42 versus 61 min in the over-65 age group, and women at 49 versus 73 min in the over-65 group. Despite these differences, dosing guidelines are the same based on age and sex for gemcitabine. Toxicities primarily include neutropenia and thrombocytopenia. Dosing modifications for hepatic and renal dysfunction have been reported [9]. Gemcitabine as a single agent displays minimal toxicity in older patients [139].

Pemetrexed
Pemetrexed is primarily excreted unchanged in the urine (70–90% in the first 24 h). It is contraindicated in patients with CrCl <45 ml/min. In patients with impaired renal function, pemetrexed plasma clearance positively correlated with GFR, which resulted in increased drug exposures. Pemetrexed 600 mg/m^2 was well tolerated (with vitamin supplementation) in patients with GFR >80 ml/min. In patients with GFR 40–79 ml/min, a dose of 500 mg/m^2 along with vitamin supplementation was tolerated [11]. Further studies are needed to determine dosing in renally impaired patients.

Camptothecins

Topotecan
Topotecan is a topoisomerase I inhibitor approved for the treatment of recurrent or refractory ovarian cancer and small cell lung cancer, and it has activity in myelodysplastic syndromes and acute myeloid leukemia. Topotecan renal clearance accounts for 30% of its elimination and it has a half-life of 3 h. A large interindividual variability was observed, with clearance varying from 9.1 to 42.51 per hour (mean 21.0). Topotecan clearance was related to serum creatinine level, and age [140]. Dose adjustments are required in patients with moderate renal impairment. Severe myelosuppression can occur if dose adjustments are not made. A specific dose modification based on CrCl has been recommended, particularly for older patients [141]. A review of patients with small cell lung cancer showed no difference in efficacy and minimal toxicity differences in patients 65 years and older compared with younger patients [142].

Irinotecan
Irinotecan is a topoisomerase I inhibitor approved for the treatment of metastatic colorectal cancer alone or in combination with 5-FU and leucovorin. It has activity in glioblastoma multiforme, non-small cell and small cell lung cancer, and gastric, esophageal, and pancreatic cancer. It can be given as a weekly and every-3-week dose [143, 144]. The weekly and once-every-3-week regimen showed similar efficacy and quality of life. Patients aged 70 years or older independently predicted occurrence of grade 3/4 diarrhea. Treatment with the every-3-week schedule was associated with a lower rate of grade 3/4 diarrhea [144]. SN-38, the major metabolite of irinotecan, is approximately 1,000 times more potent than the parent compound. The major toxicity of irinotecan therapy is delayed diarrhea and myelosuppression. Late diarrhea may be caused by intestinal accumulation of SN-38. The biliary concentration of SN-38 may be predictive of gastrointestinal toxicity, leading to the proposal of a biliary index as a surrogate measure to predict the severity of diarrhea [145]. Delayed diarrhea was increased in patients with advanced age. Pharmacokinetic parameters, such as mean irinotecan, SN-38, SN-38G, C_{max}, AUC_{0-24}, and biliary index values in patients 65 years or older, were within 3% of those in younger patients. In addition, response rates do not vary based on age [146]. It is recommended that patients over the age of 70 years, patients with prior pelvic irradiation, or poor performance status start at reduced doses [143].

Etoposide
Etoposide is a topoisomerase II inhibitor used in the treatment of refractory non-Hodgkin's lymphoma, lung cancer, germ cell tumors, and a multitude of other malignancies. It is typically given through the intravenous route, although oral therapy is also used. Oral therapy occasionally poses problems with oral absorption and

tolerance [147]. Etoposide displays bi- or triphasic pharmacokinetic characteristics with an initial half-life of 0.6–2 h (mean 0.25–2.5), and a terminal half-life of 5.3–10.8 h (mean 2.9–19). Etoposide absorption is highly variable estimated at 50%, but ranging from 25 to 75% [136, 148]. Impaired renal function leads to a decrease in drug clearance rates. Increasing age has been correlated to increased free etoposide concentrations during oral therapy correlating with leucopenia [149]. Poor performance status may place older patients at higher risk for grade 4 dose-limiting toxicities such as myelosuppression and mucositis [149]. Etoposide is eliminated to some degree via hepatic cytochrome P450 metabolism, but dosage adjustments based on liver dysfunction are controversial. The pharmacokinetics of oral etoposide in patients with liver dysfunction does not differ from patients with normal liver function [150].

Conclusion

The data presented will hopefully be able to aid clinicians in the treatment of elderly patients. Unfortunately, prospective data, particularly pharmacokinetic data, correlated with patient's functional status and clinical status does not exist. Particularly for those patients aged 80 years and older, extrapolation and most importantly, good clinical judgment are an absolute necessity. In general, age-related differences in pharmacokinetics have been demonstrated on a consistent basis. Pharmacokinetic changes that are seen are usually a reflection of end-organ dysfunction (hepatic, renal), hypoalbuminemia and anemia. The more important clinical issue is the increased toxicity that is seen particularly in those patients with poor function. Also, there is data which already exists from completed clinical trials which has never undergone an analysis by age. This situation needs to be remedied by a re-analysis and journal editors insisting that submitted publications include an age-related analysis where appropriate. Clinical trials evaluating and defining the treatment needs and the goals of therapy in elderly cancer patients are being performed. Methods for identifying high-risk individuals for developing side effects from chemotherapy are being developed. Chemotherapy approaches for several common malignancies, both in the adjuvant setting and for metastatic disease, are changing rapidly at this time. Optimizing therapeutic strategies for cancer patients who are over 65 years of age remains a challenge. Choosing the correct regimen and dose for the older patient can be extremely difficult as there are no accepted algorithms to guide management decisions in this patient group. Older cancer patients who have an adequate performance status and functional status and a reasonable life expectancy should receive the same therapies as younger patients. For those older patients with a poor performance status or functional status, single-agent reduced-dose chemotherapy options and non-chemotherapeutic approaches should be considered, together with palliative and supportive care options. Pegfilgrastim and filgrastrim can reduce the incidence of neutropenia and its sequelae [3]. The effectiveness of growth factor support has often made non-hematologic toxicity dose limiting. The National Comprehensive Cancer Network has published Senior Adult Oncology guidelines, which can greatly aid the physicians treating [151]. Investigators need to be encouraged to developed appropriate clinical trials for older patients which will be acceptable to these vulnerable individuals and their families.

References

1 Hutchins LF, Unger JM, Crowley JJ, et al: Underrepresentation of patients 65 years of age or older in cancer treatment trials. N Engl J Med 1999;341:2061–2067.
2 Talarico L, Chen G, Pazdur R: Enrollment of elderly patients in clinical trials for cancer drug registration: a 7-year experience by the US Food and Drug Administration. J Clin Oncol 2004;22:4626–4631.
3 Smith TJ, Khatcheressian J, Lyman GH, et al: 2006 update of recommendations for the use of white blood cell growth factors: an evidence-based clinical practice guideline. J Clin Oncol 2006;24:3187–3205.
4 Marx GM, Blake GM, Galani E, et al: Evaluation of the Cockroft-Gault, Jelliffe and Wright formulae in estimating renal function in elderly cancer patients. Ann Oncol 2004;15:291–295.
5 Swedko PJ, Clark HD, Paramsothy K, et al: Serum creatinine is an inadequate screening test for renal failure in elderly patients. Arch Intern Med 2003;163:356–360.
6 Levey AS, Coresh J, Greene T, et al: Using standardized serum creatinine values in the modification of diet in renal disease study equation for estimating glomerular filtration rate. Ann Intern Med 2006;145:247–254.
7 Verhave JC, Fesler P, Ribstein J, et al: Estimation of renal function in subjects with normal serum creatinine levels: influence of age and body mass index. Am J Kidney Dis 2005;46:233–241.
8 Venook AP, Enders Klein C, Fleming G, et al: A phase I and pharmacokinetic study of irinotecan in patients with hepatic or renal dysfunction or with prior pelvic radiation: CALGB 9863. Ann Oncol 2003;14:1783–1790.
9 Venook AP, Egorin MJ, Rosner GL, et al: Phase I and pharmacokinetic trial of gemcitabine in patients with hepatic or renal dysfunction: Cancer and Leukemia Group B 9565. J Clin Oncol 2000;18:2780–2787.
10 Venook AP, Egorin MJ, Rosner GL, et al: Phase I and pharmacokinetic trial of paclitaxel in patients with hepatic dysfunction: Cancer and Leukemia Group B 9264. J Clin Oncol 1998;16:1811–1819.
11 Mita AC, Sweeney CJ, Baker SD, et al: Phase I and pharmacokinetic study of pemetrexed administered every 3 weeks to advanced cancer patients with normal and impaired renal function. J Clin Oncol 2006;24:552–562.
12 Lichtman SM, Wildiers H, Chatelut E, et al: International Society of Geriatric Oncology Chemotherapy Taskforce: Evaluation of chemotherapy in older patients – an analysis of the medical literature. J Clin Oncol 2007;25:1832–1843.
13 Shah RR: Drug development and use in the elderly: search for the right dose and dosing regimen (parts I & II). Br J Clin Pharmacol 2004;58:452–469.
14 Tew KD, Colvin OM, Chabner BA: Alkylating agents; in Chabner BA, Longo DL (eds): Cancer Chemotherapy and Biotherapy: Principles and Practice, ed 3. Philadelphia, Lippincott-Raven, 2001, pp 373–414.
15 Reece PA, Hill HS, Green RM, et al: Renal clearance and protein binding of melphalan in patients with cancer. Cancer Chemother Pharmacol 1988;22:348–352.
16 Adair CG, McElnay JC: The effect of dietary amino acids on the gastrointestinal absorption of melphalan and chlorambucil. Cancer Chemother Pharmacol 1987;19:343–346.
17 Vigneau C, Ardiet C, Bret M, et al: Intermediate-dose (25 mg/m^2) intravenous melphalan for multiple myeloma with renal failure. J Nephrol 2002;15:684–689.
18 Kergueris MF, Milpied N, Moreau P, et al: Pharmacokinetics of high-dose melphalan in adults: influence of renal function. Anticancer Res 1994;14:2379–2382.
19 Tricot G, Alberts DS, Johnson C, et al: Safety of autotransplants with high-dose melphalan in renal failure: a pharmacokinetic and toxicity study. Clin Cancer Res 1996;2:947–952.

20 El Cheikh J, Kfoury E, Calmels B, et al: Age at transplantation and outcome after autologous stem cell transplantation in elderly patients with multiple myeloma. Hematol Oncol Stem Cell Ther 2011; 4:30–36.
21 Qazilbash MH, Saliba RM, Hosing C, et al: Autologous stem cell transplantation is safe and feasible in elderly patients with multiple myeloma. Bone Marrow Transplant 2007;39:279–283.
22 Klepin HD, Hurd DD: Autologous transplantation in elderly patients with multiple myeloma: are we asking the right questions? Bone Marrow Transplant 2006;38:585–592.
23 Jantunen E, Kuittinen T, Penttila K, et al: High-dose melphalan (200 mg/m^2) supported by autologous stem cell transplantation is safe and effective in elderly (> or = 65 years) myeloma patients: comparison with younger patients treated on the same protocol. Bone Marrow Transplant 2006;37:917–922.
24 Sirohi B, Powles R, Kulkarni S, et al: Glomerular filtration rate prior to high-dose melphalan 200 mg/m^2 as a surrogate marker of outcome in patients with myeloma. Br J Cancer 2001;85:325–332.
25 Facon T, Mary JY, Pegourie B, et al: Dexamethasone-based regimens versus melphalan-prednisone for elderly multiple myeloma patients ineligible for high-dose therapy. Blood 2006;107:1292–1298.
26 Mateos MV, San-Miguel J: Treatment of newly diagnosed myeloma in patients not eligible for transplantation. Curr Hematol Malig Rep 2011;6: 113–119.
27 Mahindra A, Laubach J, Raje N, et al: Latest advances and current challenges in the treatment of multiple myeloma. Nat Rev Clin Oncol 2012;9: 135–143.
28 Moore MJ: Clinical pharmacokinetics of cyclophosphamide. Clin Pharmacokinet 1991;20:194–208.
29 Beex LV, Hermus AR, Pieters GF, et al: Dose intensity of chemotherapy with cyclophosphamide, methotrexate and 5-fluorouracil in the elderly with advanced breast cancer. Eur J Cancer 1992;28: 686–690.
30 Dees EC, O'Reilly S, Goodman SN, et al: A prospective pharmacologic evaluation of age-related toxicity of adjuvant chemotherapy in women with breast cancer. Cancer Invest 2000;18:521–529.
31 Friedberg JW, Cohen P, Chen L, et al: Bendamustine in patients with rituximab-refractory indolent and transformed non-Hodgkin's lymphoma: results from a phase II multicenter, single-agent study. J Clin Oncol 2008;26:204–210.
32 Robinson KS, Williams ME, van der Jagt RH, et al: Phase II multicenter study of bendamustine plus rituximab in patients with relapsed indolent B-cell and mantle cell non-Hodgkin's lymphoma. J Clin Oncol 2008;26:4473–4479.
33 Cheson BD, Rummel MJ: Bendamustine: rebirth of an old drug. J Clin Oncol 2009;27:1492–1501.
34 Rummel MJ, Kaiser U, Balser C, et al: Bendamustine plus rituximab versus fludarabine plus rituximab in patients with relapsed follicular, indolent and mantle cell lymphomas – final results of the randomized phase III study NHL 2-2003 on behalf of the StiL (Study Group Indolent Lymphomas, Germany). ASH Annual Meeting Abstracts. Blood 2010;116:856.
35 Owen JS, Melhem M, Passarell JA, et al: Bendamustine pharmacokinetic profile and exposure-response relationships in patients with indolent non-Hodgkin's lymphoma. Cancer Chemother Pharmacol 2010;66:1039–1049.
36 Takimoto CH, Yee LK, Venzon DJ, et al: High inter- and intrapatient variation in 5-fluorouracil plasma concentrations during a prolonged drug infusion. Clin Cancer Res 1999;5:1347–1352.
37 Raghavan D, Suh T: Cancer in the elderly population: the protection racket. J Clin Oncol 2006;24: 1795–1796.
38 Stein BN, Petrelli NJ, Douglass HO, et al: Age and sex are independent predictors of 5-fluorouracil toxicity. Analysis of a large-scale phase III trial. Cancer 1995;75:11–17.
39 Meta-Analysis Group in Cancer: Toxicity of fluorouracil in patients with advanced colorectal cancer: effect of administration schedule and prognostic factors. J Clin Oncol 1998;16:3537–3541.
40 Sargent DJ, Goldberg RM, Jacobson SD, et al: A pooled analysis of adjuvant chemotherapy for resected colon cancer in elderly patients. N Engl J Med 2001;345:1091–1097.
41 Delea TE, Vera-Llonch M, Edelsberg JS, et al: The incidence and cost of hospitalization for 5-FU toxicity among Medicare beneficiaries with metastatic colorectal cancer. Value Health 2002;5:35–43.
42 Goldberg RM, Tabah-Fisch I, Bleiberg H, et al: Pooled analysis of safety and efficacy of oxaliplatin plus fluorouracil/leucovorin administered bimonthly in elderly patients with colorectal cancer. J Clin Oncol 2006;24:4085–4091.
43 Haller DG, Catalano PJ, Macdonald JS, et al: Phase III study of fluorouracil, leucovorin, and levamisole in high-risk stage II and III colon cancer: final report of Intergroup 0089. J Clin Oncol 2005; 23:8671–8678.

44 Schrag D, Cramer LD, Bach PB, et al: Age and adjuvant chemotherapy use after surgery for stage III colon cancer. J Natl Cancer Inst 2001;93:850–857.

45 Folprecht G, Cunningham D, Ross P, et al: Efficacy of 5-fluorouracil-based chemotherapy in elderly patients with metastatic colorectal cancer: a pooled analysis of clinical trials. Ann Oncol 2004;15: 1330–1338.

46 Van Cutsem E, Hoff PM, Harper P, et al: Oral capecitabine vs. intravenous 5-fluorouracil and leucovorin: integrated efficacy data and novel analyses from two large, randomised, phase III trials. Br J Cancer 2004;90:1190–1197.

47 Van Cutsem E, Twelves C, Cassidy J, et al: Oral capecitabine compared with intravenous fluorouracil plus leucovorin in patients with metastatic colorectal cancer: results of a large phase III study. J Clin Oncol 2001;19:4097–4106.

48 Twelves C: Capecitabine as first-line treatment in colorectal cancer. Pooled data from two large, phase III trials. Eur J Cancer 2002;38(suppl 2):15–20.

49 Twelves C, Wong A, Nowacki MP, et al: Capecitabine as adjuvant treatment for stage III colon cancer. N Engl J Med 2005;352:2696–2704.

50 Scheithauer W, McKendrick J, Begbie S, et al: Oral capecitabine as an alternative to intravenous 5-fluorouracil-based adjuvant therapy for colon cancer: safety results of a randomized, phase III trial. Ann Oncol 2003;14:1735–1743.

51 Hoff PM, Ansari R, Batist G, et al: Comparison of oral capecitabine versus intravenous fluorouracil plus leucovorin as first-line treatment in 605 patients with metastatic colorectal cancer: results of a randomized phase III study. J Clin Oncol 2001; 19:2282–2292.

52 Feliu J, Escudero P, Llosa F, et al: Capecitabine as first-line treatment for patients older than 70 years with metastatic colorectal cancer: an Oncopaz Cooperative Group study. J Clin Oncol 2005;23: 3104–3111.

53 Sharma R, Rivory L, Beale P, et al: A phase II study of fixed-dose capecitabine and assessment of predictors of toxicity in patients with advanced/metastatic colorectal cancer. Br J Cancer 2006;94:964–968.

54 Cassidy J, Twelves C, Van Cutsem E, et al: First-line oral capecitabine therapy in metastatic colorectal cancer: a favorable safety profile compared with intravenous 5-fluorouracil/leucovorin. Ann Oncol 2002;13:566–575.

55 Gajria D, Gonzalez J, Feigin K, et al: Phase II trial of a novel capecitabine dosing schedule in combination with lapatinib for the treatment of patients with HER2-positive metastatic breast cancer. Breast Cancer Res Treat 2011;131:111–116.

56 Gajria D, Feigin K, Tan LK, et al: Phase 2 trial of a novel capecitabine dosing schedule in combination with bevacizumab for patients with metastatic breast cancer. Cancer 2011;117:4125–4131.

57 Traina TA, Theodoulou M, Feigin K, et al: Phase I study of a novel capecitabine schedule based on the Norton-Simon mathematical model in patients with metastatic breast cancer. J Clin Oncol 2008;26: 1797–1802.

58 Camidge R, Reigner B, Cassidy J, et al: Significant effect of capecitabine on the pharmacokinetics and pharmacodynamics of warfarin in patients with cancer. J Clin Oncol 2005;23:4719–4725.

59 Massari C, Brienza S, Rotarski M, et al: Pharmacokinetics of oxaliplatin in patients with normal versus impaired renal function. Cancer Chemother Pharmacol 2000;45:157–164.

60 Takimoto CH, Remick SC, Sharma S, et al: Dose-escalating and pharmacological study of oxaliplatin in adult cancer patients with impaired renal function: a National Cancer Institute Organ Dysfunction Working Group Study. J Clin Oncol 2003;21: 2664–2672.

61 Graham MA, Lockwood GF, Greenslade D, et al: Clinical pharmacokinetics of oxaliplatin: a critical review. Clin Cancer Res 2000;6:1205–1218.

62 Aparicio T, Desrame J, Lecomte T, et al: Oxaliplatin- or irinotecan-based chemotherapy for metastatic colorectal cancer in the elderly. Br J Cancer 2003;89: 1439–1444.

63 Feliu J, Salud A, Escudero P, et al: XELOX (capecitabine plus oxaliplatin) as first-line treatment for elderly patients over 70 years of age with advanced colorectal cancer. Br J Cancer 2006;94: 969–975.

64 Comella P, Natale D, Farris A, et al: Capecitabine plus oxaliplatin for the first-line treatment of elderly patients with metastatic colorectal carcinoma: final results of the Southern Italy Cooperative Oncology Group Trial 0108. Cancer 2005;104: 282–289.

65 Mattioli R, Massacesi C, Recchia F, et al: High activity and reduced neurotoxicity of bifractionated oxaliplatin plus 5-fluorouracil/leucovorin for elderly patients with advanced colorectal cancer. Ann Oncol 2005;16:1147–1151.

66 Berardi R, Saladino T, Mari D, et al: Elderly patients with advanced colorectal cancer: tolerability and activity of chemotherapy. Tumori 2005;91:463–466.

67 Santini D, Graziano F, Catalano V, et al: Weekly oxaliplatin, 5-fluorouracil and folinic acid (OXALF) as first-line chemotherapy for elderly patients with advanced gastric cancer: results of a phase II trial. BMC Cancer 2006;6:125.

68 Rosati G, Cordio S, Tucci A, et al: Phase II trial of oxaliplatin and tegafur/uracil and oral folinic acid for advanced or metastatic colorectal cancer in elderly patients. Oncology 2005;69:122–129.

69 Reed E, Dabholkar M, Chabner BA: Platinum analogues; in Chabner BA, Longo DL (eds): Cancer Chemotherapy and Biotherapy: Principles and Practice, ed 2. Philadelphia, Lippincott-Raven, 1996, pp 357–378.

70 Daugaard G, Abildgaard U: Cisplatin nephrotoxicity. Cancer Chemother Pharmacol 1988;25:1–9.

71 Raj GV, Iasonos A, Herr H, et al: Formulas calculating creatinine clearance are inadequate for determining eligibility for cisplatin-based chemotherapy in bladder cancer. J Clin Oncol 2006;24:3095–30100.

72 Dooley MJ, Poole SG, Rischin D, et al: Carboplatin dosing: gender bias and inaccurate estimates of glomerular filtration rate. Eur J Cancer 2002;38:44–51.

73 Donahue A, McCune JS, Faucette S, et al: Measured versus estimated glomerular filtration rate in the Calvert equation: influence on carboplatin dosing. Cancer Chemother Pharmacol 2001;47:373–379.

74 Calvert AH, Egorin MJ: Carboplatin dosing formulae: gender bias and the use of creatinine- based methodologies. Eur J Cancer 2002;38:11–16.

75 Launay-Vacher V, Chatelut E, Lichtman S, et al: Renal insufficiency in elderly cancer patients: International Society of Geriatric Oncology clinical practice recommendations. Ann Oncol 2007;18:1314–1321.

76 Lichtman SM, Wildiers H, Launay-Vacher V, et al: International Society of Geriatric Oncology (SIOG) recommendations for the adjustment of dosing in elderly cancer patients with renal insufficiency. Eur J Cancer 2007;43:14–34.

77 Sachelarie I, Grossbard ML, Chadha M, et al: Primary systemic therapy of breast cancer. Oncologist 2006;11:574–589.

78 Wagner AD, Grothe W, Haerting J, et al: Chemotherapy in advanced gastric cancer: a systematic review and meta-analysis based on aggregate data. J Clin Oncol 2006;24:2903–2909.

79 Estey EH: General approach to, and perspectives on clinical research in, older patients with newly diagnosed acute myeloid leukemia. Semin Hematol 2006;43:89–95.

80 Gluck S: Adjuvant chemotherapy for early breast cancer: optimal use of epirubicin. Oncologist 2005;10:780–791.

81 Von Hoff DD, Rozencweig M, Piccart M: The cardiotoxicity of anticancer agents. Semin Oncol 1982;9:23–33.

82 Balducci L, Beghe C: Pharmacology of chemotherapy in the older cancer patient. Cancer Control 1999;6:466–470.

83 Rosner GL, Hargis JB, Hollis DR, et al: Relationship between toxicity and obesity in women receiving adjuvant chemotherapy for breast cancer: results from cancer and leukemia group B study 8541. J Clin Oncol 1996;14:3000–3008.

84 Callies S, de Alwis DP, Mehta A, et al: Population pharmacokinetic model for daunorubicin and daunorubicinol coadministered with zosuquidar.3HCl (LY335979). Cancer Chemother Pharmacol 2004;54:39–48.

85 Leone G, Sica S, Pagano L: Idarubicin including regimens in acute myelogenous leukemia in elderly patients. Crit Rev Oncol Hematol 1999;32:59–68.

86 Sandstrom M, Freijs A, Larsson R, et al: Lack of relationship between systemic exposure for the component drug of the fluorouracil, epirubicin, and 4-hydroxycyclophosphamide regimen in breast cancer patients. J Clin Oncol 1996;14:1581–1588.

87 Robert J, Rigal-Huguet F, Huet S, et al: Pharmacokinetics of idarubicin after oral administration in elderly leukemic patients. Leukemia 1990:4:227–229.

88 Marchiset-Leca D, Leca FR, Galeani A, et al: Pharmacokinetics and metabolism of pirarubicin in humans: correlation with pharmacodynamics. Cancer Chemother Pharmacol 1995;36:239–2343.

89 Aoki S, Tsukada N, Nomoto N, et al: Effect of pirarubicin for elderly patients with malignant lymphoma. J Exp Clin Cancer Res 1998;17:465–470.

90 Ralph LD, Thomson AH, Dobbs NA, et al: Maximum a posteriori bayesian estimation of epirubicin clearance by limited sampling. Br J Clin Pharmacol 2004;57:764–772.

91 Marchiset-Leca D, Leca FR, Galeani A, et al: A limited sampling strategy for the study of pirarubicin pharmacokinetics in humans. Cancer Chemother Pharmacol 1995;36:233–238.

92 Launay MC, Milano G, Iliadis A, et al: A limited sampling procedure for estimating adriamycin pharmacokinetics in cancer patients. Br J Cancer 1989;60:89–92.

93 Bressolle F, Ray P, Jacquet JM, et al: Bayesian estimation of doxorubicin pharmacokinetic parameters. Cancer Chemother Pharmacol 1991;29:53–60.

94 Wade JR, Kelman AW, Kerr DJ, et al: Variability in the pharmacokinetics of epirubicin: a population analysis. Cancer Chemother Pharmacol 1992;29:391–395.

95 Camaggi CM, Strocchi E, Tamassia V, et al: Pharmacokinetic studies of 4¢-epi-doxorubicin in cancer patients with normal and impaired renal function and with hepatic metastases. Cancer Treat Rep 1982;66:1819–1824.
96 Camaggi CM, Strocchi E, Martoni A, et al: Epirubicin plasma and blood pharmacokinetics after single intravenous bolus in advanced cancer patients. Drugs Exp Clin Res 1985;11:285–294.
97 Twelves CJ, Dobbs NA, Michael Y, et al: Clinical pharmacokinetics of epirubicin: the importance of liver biochemistry tests. Br J Cancer 1992;66: 765–769.
98 Jakobsen P, Bastholt L, Dalmark M, et al: A randomized study of epirubicin at four different dose levels in advanced breast cancer. Feasibility of myelotoxicity prediction through single blood-sample measurement. Cancer Chemother Pharmacol 1991;28: 465–469.
99 Ralph LD, Thomson AH, Dobbs NA, et al: A population model of epirubicin pharmacokinetics and application to dosage guidelines. Cancer Chemother Pharmacol 2003;52:34–40.
100 Safra T, Muggia F, Jeffers S, et al: Pegylated liposomal doxorubicin (Doxil): reduced clinical cardiotoxicity in patients reaching or exceeding cumulative doses of 500 mg/m^2. Ann Oncol 2000;11:1029–1033.
101 Zaja F, Tomadini V, Zaccaria A, et al: CHOP-rituximab with pegylated liposomal doxorubicin for the treatment of elderly patients with diffuse large B-cell lymphoma. Leuk Lymphoma 2006;47: 2174–2180.
102 Garcia-Sanz R, Hernandez J, Sureda A, et al: Pegylated liposomal doxorubicin, melphalan and prednisone therapy for elderly patients with multiple myeloma. Hematol Oncol 2006;24:205–211.
103 Biganzoli L, Robert C, Alessandro M, et al: A joined analysis of two European Organization for the Research and Treatment of Cancer (EORTC) studies to evaluate the role of pegylated liposomal doxorubicin (Caelyx™) in the treatment of elderly patients with metastatic breast cancer. Crit Rev Oncol Hematol 2006;61:84–89.
104 Theodoulou M, Hudis C: Cardiac profiles of liposomal anthracyclines: greater cardiac safety versus conventional doxorubicin? Cancer 2004;100: 2052–2063.
105 O'Brien ME, Wigler N, Inbar M, et al: Reduced cardiotoxicity and comparable efficacy in a phase III trial of pegylated liposomal doxorubicin HCl (Caelyx/Doxil) versus conventional doxorubicin for first-line treatment of metastatic breast cancer. Ann Oncol 2004;15:440–449.

106 Donelli MG, Zucchetti M, Munzone E, et al: Pharmacokinetics of anticancer agents in patients with impaired liver function. Eur J Cancer 1998;34:33–46.
107 Van den Berg HW, Desai ZR, Wilson R, et al: The pharmacokinetics of vincristine in man: reduced drug clearance associated with raised serum alkaline phosphatase and dose-limited elimination. Cancer Chemother Pharmacol 1982;8:215–219.
108 Desai ZR, Van den Berg HW, Bridges JM, et al: Can severe vincristine neurotoxicity be prevented? Cancer Chemother Pharmacol 1982;8:211–214.
109 Urien S, Bree F, Breillout F, et al: Vinorelbine high-affinity binding to human platelets and lymphocytes: distribution in human blood. Cancer Chemother Pharmacol 1993;32:231–234.
110 Gauvin A, Pinguet F, Culine S, et al: Blood and plasma pharmacokinetics of vinorelbine in elderly patients with advanced metastatic cancer. Cancer Chemother Pharmacol 2002;49:48–56.
111 Robieux I, Sorio R, Borsatti E, et al: Pharmacokinetics of vinorelbine in patients with liver metastases. Clin Pharmacol Ther 1996;59:32–40.
112 Sorio R, Robieux I, Galligioni E, et al: Pharmacokinetics and tolerance of vinorelbine in elderly patients with metastatic breast cancer. Eur J Cancer 1997;33:301–303.
113 Gauvin A, Pinguet F, Culine S, et al: Bayesian estimate of vinorelbine pharmacokinetic parameters in elderly patients with advanced metastatic cancer. Clin Cancer Res 2000;6:2690–2695.
114 Wong M, Balleine RL, Blair EY, et al: Predictors of vinorelbine pharmacokinetics and pharmacodynamics in patients with cancer. J Clin Oncol 2006;24:2448–2455.
115 Sorraritchingchai S, Thongprasert S, Charoentum C, et al: Treatment of advanced non-small cell lung cancer with vinorelbine in elderly Thai patients. J Med Assoc Thai 2004;87:367–371.
116 Rossi A, Gridelli C, Gebbia V, et al: Single-agent vinorelbine as first-line chemotherapy in elderly patients with advanced breast cancer. Anticancer Res 2003;23:1657–1664.
117 Monfardini S, Aversa SM, Zoli V, et al: Vinorelbine and prednisone in frail elderly patients with intermediate-high grade non-Hodgkin's lymphomas. Ann Oncol 2005;16:1352–1358.
118 The Elderly Lung Cancer Vinorelbine Italian Study Group: Effects of vinorelbine on quality of life and survival of elderly patients with advanced non-small-cell lung cancer. J Natl Cancer Inst 1999;91: 66–72.
119 Sonnichsen DS, Relling MV: Clinical pharmacokinetics of paclitaxel. Clin Pharmacokinet 1994;27: 256–269.

120 Lichtman SM, Hollis D, Miller AA, et al: Prospective evaluation of the relationship of patient age and paclitaxel clinical pharmacology: Cancer and Leukemia Group B (CALGB 9762). J Clin Oncol 2006;24:1846–1851.

121 Smorenburg CH, ten Tije AJ, Verweij J, et al: Altered clearance of unbound paclitaxel in elderly patients with metastatic breast cancer. Eur J Cancer 2003;39:196–202.

122 Uyar D, Frasure HE, Markman M, et al: Treatment patterns by decade of life in elderly women (>/= 70 years of age) with ovarian cancer. Gynecol Oncol 2005;98:403–408.

123 Fidias P, Supko JG, Martins R, et al: A phase II study of weekly paclitaxel in elderly patients with advanced non-small cell lung cancer. Clin Cancer Res 2001;7:3942–3949.

124 Akerley W, Sikov WM, Cummings F, et al: Weekly high-dose paclitaxel in metastatic and locally advanced breast cancer: a preliminary report. Semin Oncol 1997;24(suppl 17):87–90.

125 Seidman AD: 'Will weekly work'? Seems to be so. J Clin Oncol 2005;23:5873–5874.

126 Vacca A, Ribatti D, Iurlaro M, et al: Docetaxel versus paclitaxel for antiangiogenesis. J Hematother Stem Cell Res 2002;11:103–118.

127 Lichtman SM, Hurria A, Cirrincione CT, et al: Paclitaxel efficacy and toxicity in older women with metastatic breast cancer: combined analysis of CALGB 9342 and 9840. Ann Oncol 2012;23:632–638.

128 Tew WP, Java J, Chi D, et al: Treatment outcomes for older women with advanced ovarian cancer: results from a phase III clinical trial (GOG182). ASCO Meet Abstr 2010;28:5030.

129 Hirth J, Watkins PB, Strawderman M, et al: The effect of an individual's cytochrome CYP3A4 activity on docetaxel clearance. Clin Cancer Res 2000;6:1255–1258.

130 Extermann M: Pharmacokinetics of weekly docetaxel in elderly patients: how well can it be predicted? Personal communication, 2004.

131 Hainsworth JD, Burris HA 3rd, Yardley DA, et al: Weekly docetaxel in the treatment of elderly patients with advanced breast cancer: a Minnie Pearl Cancer Research Network phase II trial. J Clin Oncol 2001;19:3500–3505.

132 Massacesi C, Marcucci F, Boccetti T, et al: Low dose-intensity docetaxel in the treatment of pretreated elderly patients with metastatic breast cancer. J Exp Clin Cancer Res 2005;24:43–48.

133 Maisano R, Mare M, Caristi N, et al: A modified weekly docetaxel schedule as first-line chemotherapy in elderly metastatic breast cancer: a safety study. J Chemother 2005;17:242–246.

134 Tannock IF, de Wit R, Berry WR, et al: Docetaxel plus prednisone or mitoxantrone plus prednisone for advanced prostate cancer. N Engl J Med 2004;351:1502–1512.

135 Lichtman SM, Etcubanas E, Budman DR, et al: The pharmacokinetics and pharmacodynamics of fludarabine phosphate in patients with renal impairment: a prospective dose adjustment study. Cancer Invest 2002;20:904–913.

136 McEvoy G: AHFS 2000. Drug Information. Bethesda, American Society of Health System Pharmacists, 2000.

137 Martell RE, Peterson BL, Cohen HJ, et al: Analysis of age, estimated creatinine clearance and pretreatment hematologic parameters as predictors of fludarabine toxicity in patients treated for chronic lymphocytic leukemia: a CALGB (9011) coordinated Intergroup study. Cancer Chemother Pharmacol 2002;50:37–45.

138 Launay-Vacher V, Karie S, Deray G: GPR® Anticancéreux. Guide de prescription des médicaments chez le patient insuffisant rénal, ed 3. Paris, Méditions International, 2005.

139 Shepherd FA, Abratt RP, Anderson H, et al: Gemcitabine in the treatment of elderly patients with advanced non-small cell lung cancer. Semin Oncol 1997;24(suppl 7):S50–S55.

140 Montazeri A, Boucaud M, Lokiec F, et al: Population pharmacokinetics of topotecan: intraindividual variability in total drug. Cancer Chemother Pharmacol 2000;46:375–381.

141 O'Reilly S, Armstrong DK, Grochow LB: Life-threatening myelosuppression in patients with occult renal impairment receiving topotecan (letter). Gynecol Oncol 1997;67:329–330.

142 Garst J, Buller R, Lane S, et al: Topotecan in the treatment of elderly patients with relapsed small-cell lung cancer. Clin Lung Cancer 2005;7:190–196.

143 Rougier P, Van Cutsem E, Bajetta E, et al: Randomised trial of irinotecan versus fluorouracil by continuous infusion after fluorouracil failure in patients with metastatic colorectal cancer Lancet 1998;352:1407–1412. Erratum: Lancet 1998;352:1634.

144 Fuchs CS, Moore MR, Harker G, et al: Phase III comparison of two irinotecan dosing regimens in second-line therapy of metastatic colorectal cancer. J Clin Oncol 2003;21:807–814.

145 Mick R, Gupta E, Vokes EE, et al: Limited-sampling models for irinotecan pharmacokinetics-pharmacodynamics: prediction of biliary index and intestinal toxicity. J Clin Oncol 196;14:2012–2019.

146 Rothenberg ML, Cox JV, DeVore RF, et al: A multicenter, phase II trial of weekly irinotecan (CPT-11) in patients with previously treated colorectal carcinoma. Cancer 1999;85:786–795.
147 Souhami RL, Spiro SG, Rudd RM, et al: Five-day oral etoposide treatment for advanced small-cell lung cancer: randomized comparison with intravenous chemotherapy. J Natl Cancer Inst 1997;89:577–580.
148 Dorr RT, Von Hoff DD: Cancer Chemotherapy Handbook, ed 2. Norwalk, Appleton & Lange, 1994.
149 Miller AA, Rosner GL, Ratain MJ, et al: Pharmacology of 21-day oral etoposide given in combination with intravenous cisplatin in patients with extensive-stage small cell lung cancer: a Cancer and Leukemia Group B study (CALGB 9062). Clin Cancer Res 1997;3:719–725.
150 Aita P, Robieux I, Sorio R, et al: Pharmacokinetics of oral etoposide in patients with hepatocellular carcinoma. Cancer Chemother Pharmacol 1999;43: 287–294.
151 Hurria A: NCCN Clinical Practice Guidelines in Oncology. Senior Adult Oncology, Version 2, 2011.

Stuart M. Lichtman, MD
Memorial Sloan-Kettering Cancer Center
650 Commack Road
Commack, NY 11725 (USA)
E-Mail lichtmas@mskcc.org

Surgery in Older Cancer Patients – Recent Results and New Techniques: Worth the Investment?

Barbara L. van Leeuwen[a] · Monique G. Huisman[a] · Riccardo A. Audisio[b]

[a]Department of Surgery, University Medical Center Groningen, Groningen University, Groningen, The Netherlands; [b]St. Helens Teaching Hospital, University of Liverpool, St. Helens, UK

Abstract

Recent developments in oncogeriatric surgery focus on several items – preoperative risk estimation and identification of frail patients and optimization of perioperative care. New screening tools are being evaluated and show promising results. There is increasing evidence that preoperative training of frail patients might decrease the rate of postoperative complications and increase survival. The recent trend towards individualized treatment schemes will certainly be of benefit for the elderly population. More tools are becoming available to answer the most difficult question of all, namely whether surgery is the optimal treatment in this individual frail elderly oncogeriatric patient.

Copyright © 2013 S. Karger AG, Basel

The majority of cancer patients are treated either with surgery alone or as part of a multimodality treatment regime. Although the number of elderly patients in surgical oncological practice is increasing, many questions remain about the optimal decision-making and treatment planning for the oncogeriatric patient. Over recent years there has been an increase in the number of reports on outcome after oncological surgery and tools to allow a preoperative esteem of frailty. In this chapter we discuss recent results and ways to optimize treatment in the future and also discuss general consideration in the decision-making process when considering older cancer patients for a surgical operation.

Preoperative Decision-Making

The first thing a surgeon is faced with in clinic is the decision whether or not to operate the patient he is confronted with. To this purpose the appreciation of the patient's health status and associated operative risks is essential, as well as an evaluation of predicted outcomes. In spite of the increasing number of older cancer patients seen in clinic, surgeons, different from anesthetists, show no routine use of assessment tools for functional status, comorbidities or geriatric syndromes as a routine part of everyday practice [1]. Several tools are now available to assist in the preoperative decision-making process.

A correct assessment of frailty is the main target: to this purpose, several frailty scales have been tested on surgical patients.

Kristjansson et al. [2] tried a slightly different approach in patients undergoing elective surgery for colorectal cancer. Using a Comprehensive Geriatric Assessment (CGA), 185 patients ≥70 years were included in this prospective study. Postoperative mortality was low (2%) but 60% of patients suffered complications (most of them severe). When a patient was defined as frail, the risk of experiencing a severe complication increased by 1.75 and the risk of experiencing delirium and anastomotic leakage increased by 4.92 and 5.37, respectively. A CGA was superior to ASA scores in predicting postoperative morbidity. The author suggested that the use of CGA allows predicting problems such as depression, malnutrition and polypharmacy, for them to be corrected and treated in order to minimize operative risks. Conducting a CGA took 20–80 min in this study.

In everyday practice, surgeons and supporting staff are often pressed for time and there is a need for quick screening tools in order to identify those patients in need for a geriatric assessment and support.

An interesting report from Asia by Tan et al. [3] showed that frailty measured by weight loss, gait speed, grip strength, physical activity and physical exhaustion (the criteria first described by Fried) was a more accurate way to predict postoperative complications for patients undergoing major colorectal surgery than ASA, comorbidity index and POSSUM score. Of the 83 patients included in this trial, 22 experienced a major complication (26.5%) but there was no postoperative mortality.

Frailty is not only predictive of postoperative complications but it also relates to the need for postoperative institutionalization [4]. After major elective surgical procedures requiring ICU admission, roughly 30% of patients over the age of 65 years are discharged to an institution. Timed Up & Go (TUG) in excess of 15 s, functional dependence, a Charlson comorbidity index of ≥3 and a hematocrit level of ≤35% are most predictive of negative outcomes. In the presence of a frail phenotype (≥6) the rate of postoperative discharge to an institution is increased to more than 80%. Also, with advancing frailty, healthcare costs during the first 6 months after colorectal surgery increase, as does the readmission rate [5].

Recently, Kwok et al. [6] published a report using a targeted risk prediction tool to accurately assess the mortality risk in elderly patients undergoing emergency colon surgery. A set of 39 selected preoperative predictors was used to retrospectively estimate the mortality risk in 1,358 emergency colectomies for patients over the age of 80 years. The predictors most significantly associated with mortality were patient's age, total functional dependence, COPD, congestive heart failure, steroid use, SIRS and a preoperative creatinine level >1.5 mg/dl. This targeted risk prediction score correctly predicted mortality 56% of the time with a specificity of 80%. As the authors state in the discussion, this tool still does not perfectly predict mortality and the question remains how useful these tools are in everyday practice. Would and should a surgeon ever decline treatment to a patient based on a predictive tool?

Outcome Reports

When discussing elderly patients and outcomes after surgery, the emphasis has usually been on short-term outcomes and survival [7, 8]. This is not without reason; surviving surgery used to be an accomplishment in itself. However, in past decades, anesthesiological techniques and perioperative care have evolved to such an extent that early postoperative death is rare, even in the geriatric population. Reports on outcomes after major surgical interventions in the elderly population have been positive, emphasizing that for the fit elderly patient there is no limit to which surgical interventions can be effected and successfully performed, and outcomes are comparable to those in younger comparable groups [9, 10]. Several major problems remain when interpreting these seemingly positive results. Firstly, there is the problem of patient selection. As discussed above, there is no uniform definition of fit or frail, and even less uniform are the screening tools used to identify whether the patient fits into one of the two groups. Secondly, there is certainly more to life after surgery than survival. This holds true for every age category, but especially for the elderly as the remaining lifespan is shorter than in the younger age category. Preserving functional independence is key in maintaining an acceptable quality of life in older patients, yet this outcome is rarely included in surgical reports. Lawrence et al. [11] showed that a substantial group experienced protracted disability at 6 months after major abdominal operations in a group of patients aged 60 years or more. Several components of physical and mental functioning did not return to preoperative levels. One interesting example of postoperative functional decline is postoperative cognitive dysfunction (POCD). This phenomenon may affect several aspects of cognitive functioning such as memory and concentration and occurs in patients of all ages. In contrast to what is generally believed, knowledge of the incidence and impact of POCD on quality of life is limited [12]. The definition of POCD in the literature is not uniform, and there are no standardized diagnostic criteria. Although a few studies describe its incidence in an elderly surgical population, it has been studied more extensively in a younger population and in younger patients undergoing open heart surgery requiring cardiopulmonary bypass [13, 14]. The causes of POCD are postulated to be multifactorial, but there is increasing evidence that the inflammatory response caused by the surgical procedure plays a role [15, 16]. A relation between POCD and the development of Alzheimer's disease has been suggested, but so far solid evidence is lacking [17, 18]. The older brain has a reduced potential for recovery compared to the younger brain, and it is therefore to be expected that postoperative cognitive decline in the elderly patient will have major implications in terms of loss of independent functioning and quality of life. Part of our elderly population is only just able to function independently preoperatively, any functional postoperative loss will go hand in hand with increased consumption of care and increased costs.

A factor closely related with POCD is postoperative delirium. This acute cognitive complication is rarely recorded and seldom reported in the surgical literature.

A wide range of estimates of prevalence for postoperative delirium is reported, depending on the type of surgical procedure. It is estimated to affect 13–33% of patients undergoing elective abdominal aneurysm surgery [18, 19] and up to 60% of patients undergoing hip surgery [20]. Frail elderly are at increased risk of delirium with an incidence of up to 60% [21]. Although all elderly patients may be at some risk for the development of delirium, it is possible to identify patients at highest risk preoperatively and focus interventions on this group [22]. This is especially interesting as postoperative delirium is predictive of the development of long-term POCD.

Long-term survival is seldom reported among outcomes after major surgical procedures in elderly patients. Rutten et al. [23] showed that, especially in the older patient categories (≥75 years), the occurrence of complications after rectal surgery is associated with a higher postoperative mortality even at 6 months postoperatively. They go as far as to recommend non-surgical treatment for the frail elderly patient with rectal cancer. Similarly, Legner et al. [24] showed that postoperative complications after abdominopelvic surgery increase the rate of discharge to an institutional care facility for elderly patients. Both 30-day and 1-year mortality were increased in this patient group to 4.3 and 22.2%, respectively. These potential risks of a surgical intervention require more research, and surgeons treating patients in the older age groups should be made aware of this risk when consented.

Postoperative Complications

There is an interesting link between inflammation, age and cancer. Not only does aging go hand in hand with inflammation, but many comorbidities seen in the aging patient are associated with systemic inflammation such as diabetes, arthritis and atherosclerosis [25, 26]. Chronic inflammation is also associated with the development of cancer. Viewed from this perspective, it is interesting that elderly patients who suffer from a postoperative complication are more likely to either die from these complications or suffer long-term functional loss. Typical postoperative problems occurring in the geriatric population are delirium, urinary tract infections or incontinence, pneumonia and cardiovascular complications [27]. The treatment of postoperative pain is responsible for further complications in the elderly. Not only is pain differently perceived and reported from the younger group and therefore often undertreated, but elderly patients also react differently to pain treatment and benzodiazepines. Unfortunately, both the level of pain and prescribed medication are associated with an increased risk of developing postoperative delirium [28].

Several studies have recently explored the association between surgery, inflammation and age. Preoperative biomarkers such as CRP, IL-6 and TNF-α associate to frailty; higher levels of preoperative CRP and IL-6 also associate to an increased occurrence of severe postoperative complications. Bautmans et al. [29] found that older age was related to higher surgery-induced levels of IL-6 at the second and fourth day following elective abdominal surgery and worse self-perceived fatigue and muscle endurance [30]. This reduced muscle strength makes elderly patients more susceptible to persistent functional decline after major surgery.

Alternatives to Surgery

Technically speaking, there is no difference between the surgical removal of a solid tumor in an octogenarian or a 30-year-old patient. The occurrence of atherosclerosis might make resection more difficult; on the other hand, the softness of tissues can make the resection easier. The response to the operation, however, may be extremely different, depending on the age and frailty group.

In view of the above, the Hippocratic oath 'first do no harm' seems perfectly applicable to the elderly surgical population. Containing the harm by limiting the surgical intervention, whilst maintaining oncological principles (i.e. still aiming at a radical resection of the tumor), appears to be a logical school of thought when facing doubts about the treatment choice. And this is exactly where the heart of the problem is. How do we decide which patient to operate on and which to deny a risky but possibly life-saving procedure? It has been reported that declining standard breast surgery (including lymph node evaluation) to elderly women (even the octogenarians) substantially decreases breast cancer survival [31, 32]. As previously mentioned for the treatment of rectal cancer in frail elderly patients, surgically induced negative short-term outcomes may be too high to justify surgery. An interesting alternative to surgery for the treatment of patients with rectal tumors is chemoradiation only [33] with a substantial proportion of the patients treated in this way not showing any evidence of tumor recurrence, even after several years of follow-up.

In parallel to this approach, it has been shown that the wait-and-see approach for the surveillance of renal masses prevents overtreatment especially in the older and frail patient category [34]. The surgical removal of renal cell carcinomas <4 cm does not lead to a decrease in mortality, a fact that warrants consideration, especially in the frail elderly patient with decreased life expectancy.

Elderly people with small renal masses are up to 3.5 times more likely to have a benign lesion [35]. This group of patients can then be offered several treatment options. Surgical management is not to be neglected, whenever appropriate or feasible in all fit elderly patients, however frail individuals could be handled more conservatively. Since 50% of patients >70 years have a creatinine clearance <50 ml/min, nephron sparing is to be preferred when surgical ablation is the treatment plan [36].

Careful monitoring is an option. Meanwhile, repeated bioptic sampling is advisable, as the complications rate and the risk of seeding are negligible.

Limiting the surgical resection to part of the affected organ may also be a good alternative in the treatment of some tumors. Transanal endoscopic microsurgery for T_1 and T_2 rectal tumors is a far less invasive procedure than rectal resection in elderly frail patients [37]. For intra-abdominal tumors in general, the laparoscopic approach seems to be associated with better immune and inflammatory responses and earlier postoperative recovery. Although the evidence is scarce, this minimally invasive surgical approach may especially benefit the elderly patient [38]. In the earlier mentioned report by Kristjansson et al. [2], the complication rate after laparoscopic surgery was less then after open surgery [39]. Limited lung resections such as wedge resections for stage IA lung cancer (tumors ≤2 cm), instead of a formal lobectomy, have recently been shown not to decrease cancer-specific survival whilst causing less postoperative complications [40]. Again, this is an interesting alternative, especially for the frail elderly patient.

Every effort should be made to avoid the emergency setting which associates to doubled morbidity and mortality rates. In this context, self-expanding metal stents appear to be a safe alternative to emergency surgery for obstructive colorectal cancer [40]. They may be safely used as a bridge to surgery to avoid emergency surgery. Stents may also be a suitable alternative in the palliative setting.

Education and Training

A broad outlook of future investments and innovative surgical approaches for the management of older cancer patients should also include a note on education and training. Geriatric education is underrepresented in the medical curriculum and surgical training programs. The need for dedicated tutorials in Care of the Elderly within a curriculum in Surgical Oncology is obviously evident. Based on a recent publication by Biese et al. [40], it stands to reason that based on increased geriatric knowledge, doctors would be more likely to make appropriate decisions when working with oncogeriatric patients.

References

1 Bettelli G: Preoperative evaluation in geriatric surgery: comorbidity, functional status and pharmacological history. Minerva Anestesiol 2011;77:637–646.
2 Kristjansson SR, Nesbakken A, Jordhoy MS, et al: Comprehensive Geriatric Assessment can predict complications in elderly patients after elective surgery for colorectal cancer: a prospective observational cohort study. Crit Rev Oncol Hematol 2010;76:208–217.
3 Tan KY, Kawamura YJ, Tokomitsu A, Tang T: Assessment for frailty is useful for predicting morbidity in elderly patients undergoing colorectal cancer resection whose comorbidities are already optimized. Am J Surg 2012;204:139–143.
4 Robinson TN, Wallace JI, Wu DS, et al: Accumulated frailty characteristics predict postoperative discharge institutionalization in the geriatric patient. J Am Coll Surg 2011;213:37–44.

5 Robinson TN, Wu DS, Stiegmann GV, Moss M: Frailty predicts increased hospital and six-month healthcare cost following colorectal surgery in older adults. Am J Surg 2011;202:511–514.

6 Kwok AC, Lipsitz SR, Bader AM, Gawande AA: Are targeted preoperative risk prediction tools more powerful? A test of models for emergency colon surgery in the very elderly. J Am Coll Surg 2011;213:220–225.

7 Al Refaie WB, Parsons HM, Henderson WG, et al: Major cancer surgery in the elderly: results from the American College of Surgeons National Surgical Quality Improvement Program. Ann Surg 2010; 251:311–318.

8 Massarweh NN, Legner VJ, Symons RG, et al: Impact of advancing age on abdominal surgical outcomes. Arch Surg 2009;144:1108–1114.

9 Gardner GJ: Ovarian cancer cytoreductive surgery in the elderly. Curr Treat Options Oncol 2009;10:171–179.

10 Berry MF, Hanna J, Tong BC, et al: Risk factors for morbidity after lobectomy for lung cancer in elderly patients. Ann Thorac Surg 2009;88:1093–1099.

11 Lawrence VA, Hazuda HP, Cornell JE, et al: Functional independence after major abdominal surgery in the elderly. J Am Coll Surg 2004;199:762–772.

12 Culley DJ, Xie Z, Crosby G: General anesthetic-induced neurotoxicity: an emerging problem for the young and old? Curr Opin Anaesthesiol 2007;20:408–413.

13 Rasmussen LS: Postoperative cognitive dysfunction: incidence and prevention. Best Pract Res Clin Anaesthesiol 2006;20:315–330.

14 Stroobant N, van Nooten G, De Bacquer D, et al: Neuropsychological functioning 3–5 years after coronary artery bypass grafting: does the pump make a difference? Eur J Cardiothorac Surg 2008;34:396–401.

15 Van den Kommer TN, Dik MG, Comijs HC, et al: Homocysteine and inflammation: predictors of cognitive decline in older persons? Neurobiol Aging 2010;31:1700–1709.

16 Van Exel E, de Craen AJ, Remarque EJ, et al: Interaction of atherosclerosis and inflammation in elderly subjects with poor cognitive function. Neurology 2003;61:1695–1701.

17 Hu Z, Ou Y, Duan K, Jiang X: Inflammation: a bridge between postoperative cognitive dysfunction and Alzheimer's disease. Med Hypotheses 2010;74:722–724.

18 Ansaloni L, Catena F, Chattat R, Fortuna D, et al: Risk factors and incidence of postoperative delirium in elderly patients after elective and emergency surgery. Br J Surg 2010;97:273–280.

19 Benoit AG, Campbell BI, Tanner JR, et al: Risk factors and prevalence of perioperative cognitive dysfunction in abdominal aneurysm patients. J Vasc Surg 2005;42:884–890.

20 Marcantonio ER, Goldman L, Orav EJ, et al: The association of intraoperative factors with the development of postoperative delirium. Am J Med 1998;105:380–384.

21 Francis J, Martin D, Kapoor WN: A prospective study of delirium in hospitalized elderly. JAMA 1990;263:1097–1101.

22 Beliveau MM, Multach M: Perioperative care for the elderly patient. Med Clin North Am 2003;87:273–289.

23 Rutten HJ, den Dulk M, Lemmens VE, et al: Controversies of total mesorectal excision for rectal cancer in elderly patients. Lancet Oncol 2008;9:494–501.

24 Legner VJ, Massarweh NN, Symons RG, et al: The significance of discharge to skilled care after abdominopelvic surgery in older adults. Ann Surg 2009;249:250–255.

25 Provinciali M, Barucca A, Cardelli M, et al: Inflammation, aging, and cancer vaccines. Biogerontology 2010;11:615–626.

26 Cicerchia M, Ceci M, Locatelli C, et al: Geriatric syndromes in perioperative elderly cancer patients. Surg Oncol 2010;19:131–139.

27 Vaurio LE, Sands LP, Wang Y, et al: Postoperative delirium: the importance of pain and pain management. Anesth Analg 2006;102:1267–1273.

28 Ronning B, Wyller TB, Seljeflot I, et al: Frailty measures, inflammatory biomarkers and post-operative complications in older surgical patients. Age Ageing 2010;39:758–761.

29 Bautmans I, Njemini R, De Backer J, et al: Surgery-induced inflammation in relation to age, muscle endurance, and self-perceived fatigue. J Gerontol A Biol Sci Med Sci 2010;65:266–273.

30 Owusu C, Lash TL, Silliman RA: Effectiveness of adjuvant tamoxifen therapy among older women with early stage breast cancer. Breast J 2007;13:374–382.

31 Bouchardy C, Rapiti E, Blagojevic S, et al: Older female cancer patients: importance, causes, and consequences of undertreatment. J Clin Oncol 2007;25:1858–1869.

32 Habr-Gama A, Perez RO: Non-operative management of rectal cancer after neoadjuvant chemoradiation. Br J Surg 2009;96:125–127.

33 Volpe A: The role of surveillance in the management of small renal masses. ScientificWorldJournal 2007;7:860–868.

34 Rendon RA, Stanietzky N, Panzarella T, et al: The natural history of small renal masses. J Urol 2000;164:1143–1147.

35 Duncan L, Heathcote J, Djurdjev O, Levin A: Screening for renal disease using serum creatinine: who are we missing? Nephrol Dial Transplant 2001;16:1042–1046.

36 Baatrup G, Breum B, Qvist N, et al: Transanal endoscopic microsurgery in 143 consecutive patients with rectal adenocarcinoma: results from a Danish multicenter study. Colorectal Dis 2009;11:270–275.

37 Tei M, Ikeda M, Haraguchi N, et al: Postoperative complications in elderly patients with colorectal cancer: comparison of open and laparoscopic surgical procedures. Surg Laparosc Endosc Percutan Tech 2009;19:488–492.

38 Wisnivesky JP, Henschke CI, Swanson S, et al: Limited resection for the treatment of patients with stage IA lung cancer. Ann Surg 2010;251:550–554.

39 Sebastian S, Johnston S, Geoghegan T, et al: Pooled analysis of the efficacy and safety of self-expanding metal stenting in malignant colorectal obstruction. Am J Gastroenterol 2004;99:2051–2057.

40 Biese KJ, Roberts E, LaMantia M, et al: Effect of a geriatric curriculum on emergency medicine resident attitudes, knowledge, and decision-making. Acad Emerg Med 2011;18(suppl 2):S92–S96.

Prof. Riccardo A. Audisio, MD, FRCS
St. Helens Teaching Hospital, University of Liverpool
Marshalls Cross Road
St. Helens WA9 3DA (UK)
E-Mail raudisio@doctors.org.uk

Organizing the Geriatrician/Oncologist Partnership: One Size Fits All? Practical Solutions

Holly M. Holmes[a] · Gilles Albrand[b]

[a]Department of General Internal Medicine, University of Texas MD Anderson Cancer Center, Houston, Tex., USA, and [b]Programme Lyonnais d'Onco-gériatrie (PROLOG), Hôpital Geriatrique Antoine Charial, Hospices Civils de Lyon, Francheville, France

Abstract

Cancer in elderly patients is becoming a global issue, with the aging of the population and increased incidence of cancer with aging. Older patients with cancer have unique needs that can best be addressed by the integration of geriatrics principles and oncology care. Unfortunately, the worsening shortage of oncologists and geriatricians makes the care of the older patient with cancer increasingly challenging. Practical issues to consider when creating a geriatrics/oncology partnership include the available resources in terms of interdisciplinary team members, the patient population in need, and the ability to provide primary, consultative, and/or shared care. Ultimately, creative strategies will be needed to maximize the limited availability of the geriatrician and oncologist.

Copyright © 2013 S. Karger AG, Basel

The worldwide cancer burden is increasing, in part due to the aging of the population [1]. In the United States, 21% of the population – more than 80 million people – will be over the age of 65 by the year 2050 [2]. More than half of new cancers are diagnosed in people over age 65, and more than 70% of cancer deaths occur in people 65 and older [3]. In the coming decades, the increased incidence of cancer will be primarily due to the aging population [4]. As a consequence, there will be a critical and increasing need to understand the unique problems that face older people with cancer, in order to provide more effective, safe, and patient-centered care.

There are a number of reasons why future cancer care will require more than just an expansion of our current capacity, but rather a shift towards care centered on the unique needs of the elderly population. Healthcare professionals caring for older persons with cancer will need to appreciate the differences in cancer biology and outcome in older persons. Comorbid conditions, disability, and geriatric syndromes have

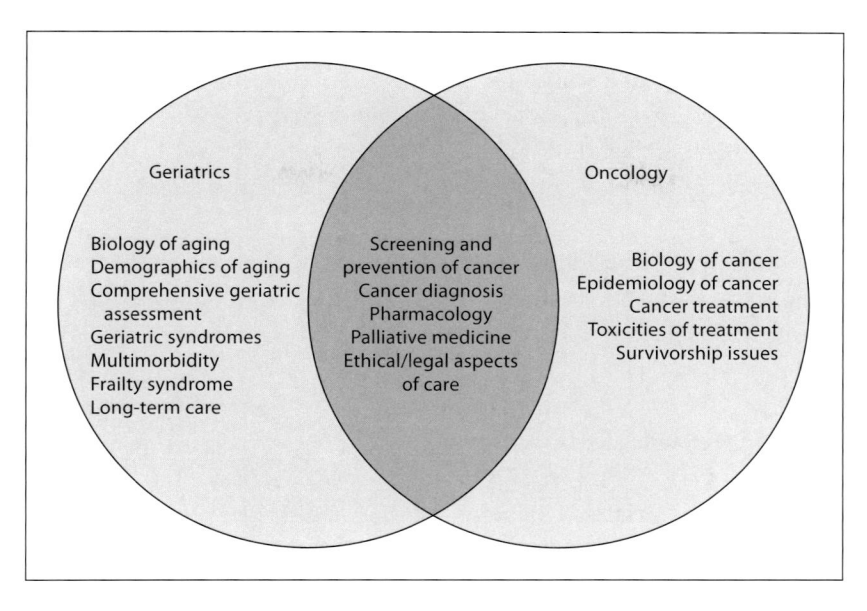

Fig. 1. Unique expertise and overlapping content areas in geriatrics and oncology.

a significant impact on cancer treatment and survivorship, and caring for older persons with cancer requires expertise in these areas (fig. 1). There are significant differences in treatment patterns for older versus younger persons with cancer [5, 6]. Furthermore, older persons may be more likely to experience toxicity from cancer therapy and thus require highly individualized treatment [7, 8]. Outcomes of treatment, including the likelihood of benefit, may be different in older patients. Finally, the preferences for outcomes that are important to older people with cancer may be different, focusing more on issues of quality of life, functional status, and independence in the community.

The Shortage of Oncologists and Geriatricians

There exists now a shortage of oncologists and particularly of geriatricians, and thus, planning for the care of older persons with cancer will require a clear strategic dialogue between these two disciplines. Currently, there are approximately 13,000 board-certified oncologists in the United States. By the year 2020, an ongoing shortfall in the number of oncologists available to care for the increasing population with cancer will result in a doubling of the demand/supply gap for cancer care [9]. Without increasing the number of fellowship spots, increasing the use of mid-level providers, or taking earlier advantage of hospice care, this shortage could be even more critical.

In geriatrics, the discrepancy is even greater. There are around 7,000 board-certified geriatricians in the United States. By the year 2050, this shortage will equate to one geriatrician for every 10,000 people in the United States 75 years and older [10]. With ongoing problems of recruitment of graduating physicians into geriatrics and poor compensation, the shortage of geriatricians will worsen in the decades to come [11].

The French situation is a little bit different with at present about 2,800 board-certified geriatricians for a total population of one-fifth of the US population, but their distribution on the territory is very heterogeneous.

Current Partnerships in Geriatrics and Oncology

The International Society of Geriatric Oncology (SIOG) 10 Priorities Initiative highlighted the global need for advancement in geriatric oncology in clinical care, education and research. Pertinent to the growth of the geriatrics-oncology partnership, integration of geriatrics and oncology into interdisciplinary care clinics is particularly needed at academic medical centers and comprehensive cancer centers. Geriatric evaluation should be incorporated into oncology care and guidelines [12].

To realistically address the burgeoning number of older people with cancer and the subsequent overwhelming number of older cancer survivors, care of the older patient with cancer will need to be shared in a collaborative model between both disciplines. Shared care models that have been proposed acknowledge the fact that the role of the primary care provider and/or geriatrician and of the oncologist is dynamic, and may depend greatly on the phase of cancer treatment and survivorship of the patient [13]. Ultimately, given the workforce shortages, both the geriatrician and the oncologist may end up assuming a much more consultative/specialist role than is currently practiced, leaving the main responsibility of care to primary care physicians. It will be fundamental that the primary care physicians insure a policy of early diagnosis of cancers to the elderly. With oncologic care being more efficient in early and localized cancers, early diagnosis will facilitate care and follow-up.

In Europe, geriatrics has been formally integrated in cancer care in models in which the geriatrician provides a consultative role that helps to inform the oncologists' decision-making [14]. The National Cancer Institute of France initiated Pilot Oncogeriatric Coordination Units (UPCOGs) to create an infrastructure for coordination of medical care between geriatricians and oncologists. In this program, geriatricians' input was used upstream or downstream of a multidisciplinary care management conference (analogous to tumor board meetings in the United States) for all patients 75 years and older with cancer. The geriatricians' roles were to screen for geriatric syndromes, provide more accurate sense of physiologic age or prognosis, and suggest preventive care. A survey of physicians involved in this program revealed some variation across different programs in the structure of care and the roles of the geriatrician and oncologist. Geriatricians were in a more supportive role, and lacked autonomy in care decision-making, and oncologists were unclear as to the geriatricians' roles [14]. In 2011, the National Cancer Institute of France pursued this action by labeling 15 Oncogeriatric Coordination Units (UCOG) whose objective is to develop partnerships between geriatrician and oncologist covering the whole national territory. The geriatricians and the oncologists are associated to equal part for the development of this new program.

In the United States, where geriatric oncology is a younger field, formal programs that integrate geriatrics and oncology do exist. In one such model, patients that meet a certain age criterion or meet screening for additional needs are seen in a separate clinical care center specifically geared towards issues of aging and cancer. Other models include geriatricians as part of the multidisciplinary cancer team, serving a supportive care role for those whose needs are identified in the oncology clinic. Another model is that of the geriatrician consultant, who may assist with patients referred from any oncology clinic to a general geriatrics practice.

Evidence of a growing collaboration is also seen in research settings. Geriatrics principles are advocated to be included in oncology trials, with the inclusion of measures and outcomes that are more important to the older patient. Geriatric assessment measures could be more routinely incorporated into the design of existing cooperative group trials [15]. Prospective cohort studies that evaluate treatment response and geriatrics specific measures could also provide a much needed evidence base for the impact of cancer treatment on more frail elderly [16].

Building a Program That Integrates Geriatrics and Oncology

Not all geriatric patients need to be seen by oncologists – indeed, though a large proportion of older patients will have cancer, many will not. Similarly, not all oncology patients need to be seen by geriatricians. Many will have geriatric syndromes such as functional loss, cognitive impairment, and falls, as well as multiple comorbidities and polypharmacy, and many will not have such problems. Thus, regardless of the model proposed for a geriatrics/oncology partnership, some common themes emerge (table 1), namely (1) the usefulness of a screening tool to identify patients who need to be seen by both oncologists and geriatricians [17, 18]; (2) the necessity of age criteria from which to select a population for both specialists; (3) the value of Comprehensive Geriatric Assessment (CGA) in patients dually evaluated by oncologists and geriatricians, and (4) the need to establish the main physician guiding the treatment plan.

Bring the Geriatrician to the Cancer Setting
In most academic settings, the geriatrician will be scarcer than the oncologist. Geriatricians may have multiple roles to play in their institution, including clinical care and teaching in inpatient, outpatient, and long-term care settings. In such situations

Table 1. Examples of geriatrics/oncology partnerships

Setting	Structure	Facilitators	Barriers
Community clinic	Geriatrician and oncologist exist in separate clinics, possibly within a hospital-affiliated system. The primary care doctor or the geriatrician likely consults the oncologist when a cancer is suspected or diagnosed.	Patients may be well known to geriatricians already, facilitating the use of CGA before cancer treatment is even considered. Common hospital system could have electronic record that could facilitate shared care.	Shortage of geriatricians in the community to provide a consultative role to the oncologist for a patient who needs CGA. Lack of communication between disciplines in a timely manner to aid with decision-making for cancer treatment.
Academic medical center	Partnership structure may be determined by the size of the geriatrics and oncology departments/centers. Consultation could occur between the geriatrician or the oncologist, depending on the referral base and entry into the hospital system.	Opportunity for standard processes to create a collaborative clinical environment. Research environment could serve as a foundation for collaboration.	Time constraints, with clinical, teaching, and research obligations of faculty members. Lack of understanding between the two disciplines about their unique expertise as well as their shared goals.
Comprehensive cancer center	Oncologists serve as a patient's primary care doctor during cancer care, and other specialists provide a consultative role. Consultation to a geriatrician could occur before, during, or after cancer care.	Use of brief screening tools (such as the CARG tool or CRASH score) to determine patients at increased toxicity risk could help the oncologist make appropriate geriatrics referrals.	High volume of older patients with cancer could overwhelm geriatrics capacity.

it may be most feasible to incorporate geriatricians into oncology care centers or to establish a strictly consultative role for the geriatrician. The optimal timing of referral to geriatricians by oncologists is unclear. In one study of geriatric assessment, the only significant difference between patients referred prior to treatment and patients referred during treatment among 65 patients ranging in age from 71 to 95 was weight loss of >10%. Otherwise, a similar number of patients were referred before compared to during treatment, and all other geriatric assessment factors were similar [19].

Bring the Oncologist to the Geriatrics Setting

Integrated management of the older cancer patient could also be achieved by bringing the oncologist (medical, surgical, or radiation) to settings in which primarily geriatric patients are managed [20]. This could occur in outpatient settings or inpatient units in which primarily geriatric patients are treated, and could even extend into nursing home consultations on the part of oncologists. Such a model of care might be necessary in a setting where geriatrics is more established, with a larger patient base, and where an oncology practice is a more recent addition to the available medical care. The advantage of such an approach is that the referral to an oncologist would occur after a CGA, providing the oncologist with valuable information on physiologic age before seeing the patient. However, such an approach would require criteria for consultation so that oncology referrals are appropriate; there could be a risk of overuse and underuse of care. In addition, the reimbursement structure for the oncologist could be unfavorable in healthcare systems such as that in the United States.

Filling the Educational Gap

Addressing the workforce shortages in both oncology and geriatrics will not be an easy task. One way to address the shortage of geriatricians despite the need for many medical disciplines to better understand the care of the older patient is to 'geriatricize' other fields, through formal, brief training programs and through education from fellowship-trained geriatricians, who will be most useful in academic clinical settings. Geriatrics has been formally integrated into medical education. The ACGME has also required geriatrics education as part of oncology fellowship training in the United States. Geriatric oncology fellowship programs have also provided the dual master clinician who can adequately care for the older patient with cancer, but more vitally, can diffuse this knowledge into both fields. Such programs have generated a small group of dual-trained, dual-certified geriatric oncologists who pave the way in terms of clinical care, education, and research, for their colleagues. In France, the choice is made towards the creation of mixed university education, oncologists-geriatricians, so that both disciplines acquire common knowledge to exchange better on the clinical, organizational plan and some clinical research.

Conclusion

Ultimately, caring for older patients with cancer will require, at a minimum, a cross-dialogue between oncology and geriatrics; geriatricians need to be oncologized and oncologists need to be geriatricized. Clinical care will increasingly require collaborative practice models with physicians, mid-level providers, and other allied health disciplines.

References

1 Jemal A, Bray F, Center MM, et al: Global cancer statistics. CA Cancer J Clin 2011;61:69–90.
2 US Census Bureau: An older and more diverse nation by midcentury. http://www.census.gov/newsroom/releases/archives/population/cb08-123.html.
3 Yancik R, Ries LA: Aging and cancer in America. Demographic and epidemiologic perspectives. Hematol Oncol Clin North Am 2000;14:17–23.
4 Smith BD, Smith GL, Hurria A, et al: Future of cancer incidence in the United States: burdens upon an aging, changing nation. J Clin Oncol 2009;27: 2758–2765.
5 Hurria A, Leung D, Trainor K, et al: Factors influencing treatment patterns of breast cancer patients age 75 and older. Crit Rev Oncol Hematol 2003;46: 121–126.
6 Wang S, Wong ML, Hamilton N, et al: Impact of age and comorbidity on non-small-cell lung cancer treatment in older veterans. J Clin Oncol 2012;30: 1447–1455.
7 Hardy D, Cormier JN, Xing Y, et al: Chemotherapy-associated toxicity in a large cohort of elderly patients with non-small cell lung cancer. J Thorac Oncol 2010;5:90–98.
8 Repetto L: Greater risks of chemotherapy toxicity in elderly patients with cancer. J Support Oncol 2003; 1(suppl 2):18–24.
9 Erikson C, Schulman S, Kosty M, Hanley A: Oncology Workforce: results of the ASCO 2007 Program Directors Survey. J Oncol Pract 2009;5:62–65.
10 ADGAP Workforce Study. http://www.adgapstudy.uc.edu/ (accessed July 2012).
11 Leipzig RM, Hall WJ, Fried LP: Treating our societal scotoma: the case for investing in geriatrics, our nation's future, and our patients. Ann Intern Med 2012;156:657–659.
12 Extermann M, Aapro M, Audisio R, et al: The SIOG 10 Priorities Initiative. 2011. http://www.siog.org.
13 Cohen HJ: A model for the shared care of elderly patients with cancer. J Am Geriatr Soc 2009; 57(suppl 2):S300–S302.
14 Sifer-Riviere L, Saint-Jean O, Gisselbrecht M, et al: What the specific tools of geriatrics and oncology can tell us about the role and status of geriatricians in a pilot geriatric oncology program. Ann Oncol 2011;22:2325–2329.
15 Hurria A: Incorporation of geriatric principles in oncology clinical trials. J Clin Oncol 2007;25: 5350–5351.
16 Mohile SG, Wildiers H: A call for observational cohort studies in geriatric oncology. J Geriatr Oncol 2012;3:291–293.
17 Bellera CA, Rainfray M, Mathoulin-Pélissier S, et al: Screening older cancer patients: first evaluation of the G-8 geriatric screening tool. Ann Oncol 2012; 23:2166–2172.
18 Mohile SG, Bylow K, Dale W, et al: A pilot study of the Vulnerable Elders Survey-13 compared with the Comprehensive Geriatric Assessment for identifying disability in older patients with prostate cancer who receive androgen ablation. Cancer 2007;109: 802–810.
19 Lazarovici C, Khodabakhshi R, Leignel D, et al: Factors leading oncologists to refer elderly cancer patients for geriatric assessment. J Geriatr Oncol 2011;2:194–199.
20 Monfardini S, Giordano G, Sandri R, Gnocchi PL, Galetti G: Bringing geriatrics into oncology or also oncology into geriatrics? Ann Oncol 2012;23:801.

Holly M. Holmes, MD
Department of General Internal Medicine
University of Texas MD Anderson Cancer Center
1515 Holcombe Blvd., Unit 1465, Houston, TX 77030 (USA)
E-Mail hholmes@mdanderson.org

Geriatric Oncology Nursing: Beyond Standard Care

Janine Overcash

The Ohio State University Comprehensive Cancer Center – Arthur G. James Cancer Hospital and Richard J. Solove Research Institute, Columbus, Ohio, USA

Abstract

Geriatric oncology nursing is a specialization that requires unique knowledge and education to care for the older person diagnosed with cancer. Understanding principles of functioning in a multidisciplinary team setting, assessment of an older patient, and cancer-related issues are central elements of the role of the geriatric oncology nurse. Additionally, education of patients and families are important in helping the older person navigate the healthcare system. The purpose of this chapter is to review the current literature in geriatric oncology nursing.

Copyright © 2013 S. Karger AG, Basel

Geriatric Oncology Nursing: Beyond Standard Care

Geriatric oncology nursing care requires patience, specialized knowledge and an interest in understanding aging as it intertwines with cancer care. Combining the principles of geriatrics and gerontology with the science of oncology nursing provides the foundation for the intricate care many older cancer patients require. Maintaining independence and quality of life of the older cancer patient despite complex diagnoses is a prime role for the geriatric oncology nurse. The geriatric oncology nurse has roles in leadership, psychosocial care, assessment and screening, physical follow-up, discharge planning and research. Combining principles associated with geriatric care such as working in a multidisciplinary team (MDT), conducting and coordinating the Comprehensive Geriatric Assessment (CGA), appreciating physical and mental decline, understanding how functional status and life expectancy relate to cancer treatment decisions with specialized oncology knowledge such as cancer treatment options, staging, and potential side effects are the essence of geriatric oncology nursing. This chapter will highlight some of the functions of the geriatric oncology nurse.

Multidisciplinary Team

The geriatric oncology nurse is a core member of the MDT; working to blur roles and professional boundaries, foster cooperation among team members and inspire professional dialogue. The integration of expertise from disciplines such as nursing, pharmacy, medicine, surgery, rehabilitation therapy, physical therapy, social work, dietary and many others who understand the needs of the older person is important to the complex care often required by older cancer patients. A role often performed by the geriatric oncology nurse is to coordinate the information provided by the MDT by inspiring team dialogue and compiling all the clinical and psychosocial information into an individualized plan of care. The nurse is the central depository for patient information for dissemination to team members, community providers, patients and families.

MDT interaction in the clinical setting is essential to providing the comprehensive care necessary to address the needs of the older cancer patient [1]. Discussion among the MDT concerning clinical impressions, social support issues and cancer treatment decisions all common examples of vital communication topics. Regular MDT meetings must occur after initiation of the plan of care in order to address potential health and/or functional status changes, social support issues that may affect cancer treatment and other events that may have impact on oncology care. Often, the geriatric oncology nurse is responsible to motivate and coordinate MDT communication and reflect all care information in the plan of care. In geriatric oncology, the MDT plan of care is a comprehensive plan that addresses physical, emotional, functional, psychosocial, and cancer-related issues [2]. Coordinating the development and ongoing maintenance of the MDT plan of care are within the scope of practice of the geriatric oncology nurse. Constant updates and changes to the plan of care are common and become a large part of the nurse's daily activities.

Teams require constant nurture to function productively. The leadership role of the geriatric oncology nurse must extend to the construction and ongoing maintenance of the MDT. Teams must be constructed with prudent forethought with respect to including the necessary disciplines (social work, dietary, physical therapy) providing adequate team training and defining specific goals and objectives. Often, team members only function as part of the geriatric oncology team during scheduled clinic times or meetings. It is important for the nurse to preserve the integrity of the team by creating an atmosphere of positive teamwork, acceptance and gratitude for participation. In addition to a positive atmosphere, the John A. Hartford Foundation suggests that teamwork requires training in order for all team members to effectively work together [3]. Team training can occur with programs such as the Geriatric Interdisciplinary Team Training program (GITT) [4] where awareness of role, communication strategies, and attitude are components of the curriculum. Team training is effective in establishing positive attitudinal change among team members [5] and addressing problems associated with discipline specific differences and cultural traditions or each profession [6]. A disciplinary split among team members associated with academic preparation, role and incorrect perceptions of role can be a barrier to effective teamwork [6]. Frequent meetings and open communication must be facilitated in order for each member to feel valued.

An essential element to the effectiveness of the team is organizational leadership. Each member of the geriatric MDT must have proper time allocation to participate in clinical practice and perform operational activities such as weekly meetings to discuss patients and other issues. Negotiating with hospital administration the necessary time requirements for each team member is an important leadership role for the nurse. Procuring protected clinical time and time for team meetings are central for the proper functioning of the MDT.

Comprehensive Geriatric Assessment

The CGA is a battery of assessment instruments used to screen older patients for problems or limitations that may go unnoticed by a general examination [7, 8]. In oncology, the CGA is used to determine cancer treatment options based on issues such as functional status, performance status and available social support [9]. The CGA provides information not often included in the traditional oncology assessment which helps predict risk [10] postoperative complications [11] and toxicity to cancer chemotherapy treatment [12]. The CGA is often performed by the MDT with each discipline conducting a different part of the assessment. The role of the geriatric oncology nurse is to orchestrate the MDT to conduct each aspect of the CGA in a timely and efficient manner, to compile the findings and arrange discussion at the regular team meetings.

The CGA addresses problems not traditionally assessed as part of oncology care [8]. Nonmalignant problems or syndromes such as falls, incontinence, dementia, and depression can be potentially identified using the CGA and must be further diagnosed or treated with a primary care provider in the community. Partnerships with community providers are necessary to maintain the continuity of care for the older patient. The treatment plan of outside providers should be discussed with the cancer MDT and considered in the cancer treatment plan. Patients who have several health limitations, considered frail and/or have multiple comorbid conditions tend to gain more benefit from the MDT approach to care [13]. Frail patients often require more services upon discharge, more comprehensive interventions and a tailored interdisciplinary plan of care to address the complexities of physical and or mental decompensation [14]. The geriatric oncology nurse is often the conduit between community providers, MDT members and patient and families.

Regular team meetings are necessary to discuss CGA results, oncology care and any specific challenges to new and established patients. Team members can become familiar with each aspect of the comprehensive care plan during the meetings and have better understanding of each MDT member's role and individual expertise. The nurse often assumes a central role during the team meetings in communicating among team members, taking note of information necessary for the community providers and providing follow-up information from previous comprehensive care plans. For inpatients, discharge planning discussions during the team meeting are critical for a smooth transition to reduce rehospitalizations up to 3 months following hospital discharge [15].

The patient and family are prime members of the MDT. Findings resulting from the CGA should be presented to the patient and family so that joint healthcare decisions can occur. Health management strategies that are not favored by the caregiver or patient tend to receive poor adherence [13, 16]. Integrating the patient and family into the decision-making process and the MDT discussions are functions of the geriatric oncology nurse. Empowering the patient and family to be vital members of the team will help develop a reasonable comprehensive plan of care that is realistic for actual implementation. For people diagnosed with cancer over the age of 80 years, family involvement in cancer treatment decisions tend to increase as compared to people who are younger [17].

Patient and Family Education

Education is important to patients and families of all ages, however older patients tend to require more medications and have multiple comorbid conditions in addition to the diagnosis and treatment of cancer [9]. The geriatric oncology nurse must work with other members of the team to educate the patient and family about medications that may be reasonable to discontinue, alter or maintain while undergoing cancer treatment. Educational needs of patients and families often focus on the cancer diagnosis, treatment, physical care, investigative tests and psychosocial needs [5]. After surgery, fear of recurrence, anxiety and physical limitations are all commonly reported problems that can be addressed with postsurgical education [18].

Other educational foci aside from cancer-related topics are important to patients and families. Orientation to the cancer facility to familiarize patients and families with the areas where treatments and clinical assessment will occur tends to reduce anxiety [1]. Cancer survivors have educational needs that surround supportive care options such as support groups, disease progression and general health [6]. For caregivers, cancer education improves notions of well-being [19], quality of life, burden of patient symptoms and task burden [20].

Patient and Family Advocate

A strong role for the geriatric oncology nurse is that of patient/family advocate. Promoting treatment decisions by coaching the patients and families to participate in the MDT discussions can result in a treatment plan consistent with the patient preferences [21]. Nurses can provide a voice to patients and family who may feel inadequate in communicating with the MDT. In terms of complementary and alternative medicine (CAM) interventions, nurses as patient advocates can help patients select CAM options patients and families may feel are important [22]. Nurses have the expertise to provide geriatric oncology education and patient advocacy that can empower patients and families to partake in the MDT discussions and feel a valuable part of the team [23].

Nursing Research in Geriatric Oncology

Nurses have many roles in the care of the older cancer patient that provide the infrastructure for evidence-based practice and clinical research. Reviewing the published literature to critically understand the most appropriate screening instruments to detect common age-related problems and identify nursing best practices in symptom management are examples of evidence-based practice which will lead to improved patient outcomes and a high quality of patient care [24].

Some examples of nurse-led research are detailed as part of the Senior Adult Oncology Program at the H. Lee Moffitt Cancer Center & Research Institute. One of the first nursing research projects addressed the issue of identifying patients who were in most need of the CGA. This project was significant in that the MDT wanted a prescreening CGA measure that would reduce patient/respondent burden for people who did not require the entire CGA and reduce clinic wait times [25, 26]. The CGA instruments that were examined in order to construct the prescreening measure were the Geriatric Depression Scale [27], the Mini-Mental State Examination [28], the Activities of Daily Living Scale [29] and the Instrumental Activities of Daily Living Scale [30]. Through the work of the MDT, the Abbreviated Comprehensive Geriatric Assessment (aCGA) and scoring cut-points were developed to address the needs of the older cancer patient.

Another example of nursing research was to understand the extent to which older people who are diagnosed with cancer experience falls and how can falls be predicted. For older people diagnosed with cancer and ongoing chemotherapy, 33% reported that they experienced a fall in 3 months prior to the interview compared to 25% of older cancer patients not receiving chemotherapy [31]. Another nurse-led research project found that older patients who reported a compromised functional status were at greater risk for falls [32]. Further investigation on the topic of falls found that the Timed Up & Go [33] was a more sensitive and specific predictor of falls compared to the Simmonds Performance Test Battery [34] and required less clinical time to administered [35].

The role of the geriatric oncology nurse as a researcher is robust in that many facets of assessment remain unexplored. Understanding how to assess the older cancer patient in a timely manner, exploring when to administer assessments (during chemotherapy, following treatment) and understanding how to integrate the findings into the comprehensive plan of care are critical elements of geriatric oncology care and well within the scope of nursing research.

Conclusions

Cancer is a disease of aging [36] and the combination of geriatric and oncology nursing science is critical to meet the needs of the growing aging population of the United States. Funding is necessary in order to provide educational opportunities to nurses who want to specialize in geriatric oncology nursing. Further support is necessary to support geriatric and oncology graduate and undergraduate curriculum. Specialized knowledge in geriatrics must be stressed in all aspects of nursing education in order to care for the demographically aging population in the United States.

References

1 Chan R, Webster J, Marquart L: Information interventions for orienting patients and their carers to cancer care facilities. Cochrane Database Syst Rev 2011;12:CD008273.
2 Overcash JA: Health needs of the older cancer patient. Constructing a comprehensive geriatric assessment. Adv Nurse Pract 2008;16:53–54, 56–58.
3 Chan R, Webster J: A national rollout of an insufficiently evaluated practice: how evidence based are our end-of-life care policies? J Palliat Med 2011;14: 802, reply 803.
4 Ling CC, Lui LY, So WK: Do educational interventions improve cancer patients' quality of life and reduce pain intensity? Quantitative systematic review. J Adv Nurs 2012;68:511–520.
5 Lei CP, Har YC, Abdullah KL: Informational needs of breast cancer patients on chemotherapy: differences between patients' and nurses' perceptions. Asian Pac J Cancer Prev 2011;12:797–802.
6 Marbach TJ, Griffie J: Patient preferences concerning treatment plans, survivorship care plans, education, and support services. Oncol Nurs Forum 2011; 38:335–342.
7 NIH: Geriatric assessment methods for clinical decision making. Natl Inst Health Consens Dev Conf Consens Statement 1987;6:1–8.
8 Overcash JA, Beckstead J, Extermann M, Cobb S: The abbreviated comprehensive geriatric assessment: a retrospective analysis. Crit Rev Oncol Hematol 2005;35:155–160.
9 Balducci L, Colloca G, Cesari M, Gambassi G: Assessment and treatment of elderly patients with cancer. Surg Oncol 2010;19:117–123.
10 Klepin HD, Geiger AM, Tooze JA, et al: The feasibility of inpatient geriatric assessment for older adults receiving induction chemotherapy for acute myelogenous leukemia. J Am Geriatr Soc 2011;59: 1837–1846.
11 Fukuse T, Satoda N, Hijiya K, Fujinaga T: Importance of a comprehensive geriatric assessment in prediction of complications following thoracic surgery in elderly patients. Chest 2005;127:886–891.
12 Freyer G, Geay JF, Touzet S, et al: Comprehensive geriatric assessment predicts tolerance to chemotherapy and survival in elderly patients with advanced ovarian carcinoma: a GINECO study. Ann Oncol 2005;16:1795–1800.
13 Esmail R, Brazil K, Lam M: Compliance with recommendations in a geriatric outreach assessment service. Age Ageing 2000;29:353–356.
14 Schonberg MA, Silliman RA, McCarthy EP, Marcantonio ER: Factors noted to affect breast cancer treatment decisions of women aged 80 and older. J Am Geriatr Soc 2012;60:538–544.
15 Legrain S, Tubach F, Bonnet-Zamponi D, et al: A new multimodal geriatric discharge-planning intervention to prevent emergency visits and rehospitalizations of older adults: the optimization of medication in AGEd multicenter randomized controlled trial. J Am Geriatr Soc 2011;59:2017–2028.

16 Maly RC, Leake B, Frank JC, et al: Implementation of consultative geriatric recommendations: the role of patient-primary care physician concordance. J Am Geriatr Soc 2002;50:1372–1380.
17 Schonberg MA, Silliman RA, McCarthy EP, Marcantonio ER: Factors noted to affect breast cancer treatment decisions of women aged 80 and older. J Am Geriatr Soc 2012;60:538–544.
18 Stephens PA, Osowski M, Fidale MS, Spagnoli C: Identifying the educational needs and concerns of newly diagnosed patients with breast cancer after surgery. Clin J Oncol Nurs 2008;12:253–258.
19 Creedle C, Leak A, Deal AM, et al: The impact of education on caregiver burden on two inpatient oncology units. J Cancer Educ 2012;27:250–256.
20 McMillan SC, Small BJ, Weitzner M, et al: Impact of coping skills intervention with family caregivers of hospice patients with cancer: a randomized clinical trial. Cancer 2006;106:214–222.
21 Tariman JD, Berry DL, Cochrane B, et al: Physician, patient, and contextual factors affecting treatment decisions in older adults with cancer and models of decision making: a literature review. Oncol Nurs Forum 2012;39:E70–E83.
22 Rojas-Cooley MT, Grant M: Complementary and alternative medicine: oncology nurses' knowledge and attitudes. Oncol Nurs Forum 2009;36:217–224.
23 Hellwig SD, Yam M, DiGiulio M: Nurse case managers' perceptions of advocacy: a phenomenological inquiry. Lippincotts Case Manag 2003;8:53–65.
24 Melnyk BM, Fineout-Overholt E, Stetler C, Allan J: Outcomes and implementation strategies from the first US Evidence-Based Practice Leadership Summit. Worldviews Evid Based Nurs 2005;2:113–121.
25 Overcash JA, Beckstead J, Extermann M, Cobb S: The abbreviated comprehensive geriatric assessment (aCGA): a retrospective analysis. Crit Rev Oncol Hematol 2005;54:129–136.
26 Overcash JA, Beckstead J, Moody L, et al: The abbreviated comprehensive geriatric assessment (aCGA) for use in the older cancer patient as a prescreen: scoring and interpretation. Crit Rev Oncol Hematol 2006;59:205–210.
27 Yesavage JA, Brink TL, Rose TL, et al: Development and validation of a geriatric depression screening scale: a preliminary report. J Psychiatr Res 1982;17:37–49.
28 Folstein M, Folstein SE, McHugh PR: 'Mini-mental state'. A practical method for grading the cognitive state of patients for the clinician. J Psychiatr Res 1975;12:189–198.
29 Katz S, Downs TD, Cash HR, Grotz RC: Progress in development of the index of ADL. Gerontologist 1970;10:20–30.
30 Lawton M, Brody EM: Assessment of older people: self-maintaining and instrumental activities of daily living. Gerontologist 1969;9:179–186.
31 Overcash JA, Beckstead J: Predicting falls in older patients using components of a comprehensive geriatric assessment. Clin J Oncol Nurs 2008;12:941–949.
32 Overcash JA: Prediction of falls in older adults with cancer: a preliminary study. Oncol Nurs Forum 2007;34:341–346.
33 Podsiadlo D, Richardson S: The timed 'Up & Go': a test of basic functional mobility for frail elderly persons. J Am Geriatr Soc1991;39:142–148.
34 Simmonds MJ: Physical function in patients with cancer: psychometric characteristics and clinical usefulness of a physical performance test battery. J Pain Symptom Manage 2001;24:404–414.
35 Overcash JA, Rivera HR Jr: Physical performance evaluation of older cancer patients: a preliminary study. Crit Rev Oncol Hematol 2008;68:233–241.
36 US Prevalence: US Estimated Prevalence counts were estimated by applying US populations to SEER 9 Limited Duration Prevalence proportions. Populations from January 2002 were based on the average of the July 2001 and July 2002 population estimates from the US Bureau of Census, 2004.

Janine Overcash, PhD, GNP-BC
The Ohio State University Comprehensive Cancer Center –
Arthur G. James Cancer Hospital and Richard J. Solove Research Institute
College of Nursing, 1585 Neil Ave., 034 Newton Hall, Columbus, OH 43210 (USA)
E-Mail janine.overcash@osumc.edu

Exercise for Older Cancer Patients: Feasible and Helpful?

Heidi D. Klepin[a] · Supriya G. Mohi e[b] · Shannon Mihalko[c]

[a]Wake Forest School of Medicine, Winston-Salem, N.C., [b]School of Medicine and Dentistry, University of Rochester Medical Center, Rochester, N.Y., and [c]Wake Forest University, Winston-Salem, N.C., USA

Abstract

Older adults are at high risk for functional decline after a cancer diagnosis. Physiologic changes of aging which negatively impact body composition, strength, and fitness increase vulnerability to the development of short- and long-term disability when stressed with cancer burden and treatments. Treatment-associated physical disability impairs quality of life, limits therapeutic options, and contributes to the social and economic burden of cancer care in the elderly. Despite this, few clinical trials capture disability as an outcome or focus on whether it can be ameliorated in this population. Exercise has multiple positive effects on physical health and well-being in non-cancer elderly populations and holds promise as a supportive care intervention to improve physical function and symptoms during and after cancer treatments. The majority of studies supporting the positive benefits of exercise among cancer survivors have been performed in younger patients. Results from limited elderly-specific trials suggest that physical activity interventions are safe and effective in older cancer survivors, with prostate cancer survivors representing the best studied cohort of older persons with cancer. Many questions remain unanswered with respect to optimal timing, mode, intensity, and delivery of exercise interventions for older patients. While available data support the potential benefit of exercise for elders with cancer, recommendations will need to be individualized to optimize participation, safety, and efficacy.

Copyright © 2013 S. Karger AG, Basel

Aging is associated with declines in physical health and well-being which can be further exacerbated by cancer burden and cancer treatment. Cancer treatments can cause both functional decline and symptoms during and after therapy that may preclude completion of optimal treatment and impair quality of life and independence. Developing and promoting interventions that improve function and minimize symptoms during receipt of cancer treatments, as well as after treatment in longer term cancer survivors, is critical for maximizing outcomes in older adults with cancer. Exercise interventions hold promise to improve physical health, well-being and, potentially, treatment tolerance for older adults. This chapter will review the rationale and evidence supporting exercise in older cancer patients and highlight special challenges in this population.

Older Adults Are at Risk for Functional Decline after a Cancer Diagnosis

Many changes associated with aging increase the risk of developing functional decline and decreased quality of life during and after cancer treatment. Older adults are particularly vulnerable to impairments in physical function. Aging is associated with changes in body composition including decreased muscle mass, strength and quality, and increased adiposity. Sarcopenia is a term used to describe the combination of low muscle mass and function (strength and performance) associated with aging [1]. Increasing age is also associated with decreased flexibility and loss of bone mass. Functional capacity reflecting cardiorespiratory fitness declines significantly with age beginning as early as the second or third decade of life. On average, patients ≥75 years of age have lost over half of the functional capacity of the cardiovascular system (defined as the maximal oxygen consumption (Vo_{2max})) [2]. Taken together, these changes in body composition, strength, flexibility, and functional capacity result in varying degrees of limitations in daily function, inactivity, and increased risks for adverse events such as falls.

In addition to changes related to physical function, older adults are at increased risk for decline in cognition and symptoms related to mood disorders. Depressive symptoms are common among older adults as are anxiety-related symptoms. These conditions can negatively impact well-being and quality of life and can also contribute to declines in physical function and increased inactivity. In summary, physiologic and psychosocial changes, and common conditions associated with aging, may decrease resilience in times of stress and increase vulnerability to adverse outcomes during and after cancer treatment.

Impact of Cancer Treatment on Physical Health and Well-Being

Physical Function
Cancer treatment may contribute to short- and long-term disability in older cancer patients. Multiple studies have demonstrated increased reported physical limitations including problems with mobility and activities of daily living among older cancer survivors compared to age-matched non-cancer controls [3–5]. This trend is reported irrespective of cancer treatments received, although the trajectory and duration of functional decline may differ significantly in each clinical scenario. For example, indolent, early stage cancers may impact function less than more aggressive or advanced stage malignancies. In addition, surgery, radiation, chemotherapy

and hormonal therapy all have differing short- and long-term side effects which may exacerbate age-associated functional declines acutely or chronically.

The short-term impact of cancer treatment on task-specific functional abilities and objective physical performance has not been well studied in older patients. One of the best studied models is in the setting of androgen deprivation therapy (ADT) for prostate cancer. Men receiving ADT demonstrate measurable declines in strength compared to age-matched patients with or without cancer after only 3 months of therapy [6]. The impact of cytotoxic chemotherapy, which can reflect a more acute stress, on physical function for older patients has not been well studied but is frequently observed in clinical practice. Multiple factors likely contribute to post-chemotherapy-related functional decline, including increased acute and chronic side effects among older adults [7], decreased physical activity during and after treatment [8], and changes in body composition. Unfortunately, oncology clinical trials to date have not routinely addressed preservation of function as an outcome of therapy. The degree to which each cancer treatment modality (surgery, chemotherapy, radiation) impacts physical function, including the trajectory of decline and recovery, has been poorly studied.

Symptoms

Cancer and its treatments have been consistently associated with symptoms which impair functional status and quality of life in both older and younger patients. Fatigue is the most common complaint among cancer patients. In one study of older cancer patients, almost all (99%) reported fatigue within a week of the assessment, with 84% reporting fatigue significant enough to interfere with their general level of activity [9]. The etiology of fatigue in this setting is multifactorial, and it is associated with global quality of life, depressive symptoms, and functional status.

The stress of a cancer diagnosis and subsequent treatments is also associated with mood disturbances including depressive symptoms, distress, and anxiety. Depression is a common symptom among older community-dwelling adults with rates increasing significantly among older adults requiring institutionalization. Older adults, however, may be at risk for under-recognition of this disorder. It is estimated that up to 1 in 4 older adults with cancer may have symptoms of depression [10]. Psychological distress may be even more common with up to 41% of older cancer patients reporting significant symptomatology [11]. Significant distress is associated with poor physical function, highlighting the link between psychological symptoms and physical disability in older adults with cancer.

Rationale for Exercise to Improve Physical Health and Well-Being

Exercise is known to have multiple positive effects which may minimize functional loss and improve quality of life in older cancer patients. The majority of data supporting the role of exercise in cancer patients is derived from studies of younger or middle-aged adults. There is a paucity of elderly-specific trials or trials which have included large proportions of older patients. Studies in younger cancer patients and in non-cancer elderly populations provide a foundation to examine the current evidence and highlight some of the challenges of extrapolating this into an elderly cancer population.

Benefits of Exercise in Non-Cancer Elderly Populations

Multiple benefits of exercise have been demonstrated among non-cancer elderly populations including those with significant comorbid conditions such as chronic pulmonary disease, cardiovascular disease, and arthritis. Exercise can improve both muscle mass and strength which can attenuate age-related declines that increase risks for future disability [12]. Exercise improves both self-reported and objective physical function such as walking speed. Improvements in strength, endurance, and balance decrease fall risk. Even among frail elders, exercise can improve physical performance and decrease self-reported disability [13]. The degree to which exercise can improve long-term independence is currently under investigation in a large randomized controlled trial. Additional health benefits include improved cardiovascular health, decreased mood disorders, and potential attenuation of cognitive decline [14, 15]. The American College of Sports Medicine and the American Heart Association Older Adults guidelines recommend a graduated program of aerobic activity, strength training, flexibility, and balance exercises for community-dwelling older adults [16]. Evidence is limited for older adults who are hospitalized or institutionalized.

Exercise for Cancer Survivors

There is substantial evidence to support the benefits of exercise on physical function and quality of life in non-elderly adults with cancer. Speck et al. [17] conducted a meta-analysis of 82 high-quality controlled clinical trials investigating physical activity interventions in cancer patients. Most of the interventions were post-treatment and focused on women with breast cancer. The average sample size was small and ranged from single digits to approximately 600 subjects with a mean of 41. Most interventions were longer than 5 weeks in duration and primarily focused on aerobic activities of a moderate to vigorous intensity delivered 3–5 times per week. No safety concerns were identified. The largest positive effects of interventions post-treatment were improvements in upper and lower body strength with moderate improvement in fatigue. A smaller effect was demonstrated for improved functional quality of life and decreased anxiety. Another meta-analysis analyzed 15 randomized exercise interventions that reported on depressive symptoms as an outcome. Exercise had a modest positive effect on depressive symptoms overall with larger effects seen if the program was supervised, located outside the home and at least 30 min in duration [18].

Consensus guidelines, such as those from the American Cancer Society, recommend adopting a physically active lifestyle during and after treatment for cancer. Guidelines are intentionally vague during active treatment, with recommendations to individualize interventions in this setting. Recommendations are more specific during the post-treatment survivorship period including ≥30 min of moderate to vigorous physical activity at least 5 days per week [19].

Exercise in Older Cancer Patients – Rationale Is Strong but Evidence Is Lacking

Elderly-specific data for exercise during and after treatment for cancer are scarce (table 1). Courneya et al. [20] reviewed 48 exercise intervention studies that provided information on age and found that almost 20% specifically excluded older adults from participation. Only two studies enrolled patients over the age of 75 years. Most exercise interventions have enrolled primarily middle-aged patients with a mean age of approximately 50 years and excluded patients with significant comorbidity.

The first large study to investigate physical activity among older adults specifically used survey methods to examine the relationship between exercise and self-reported physical functioning among 688 older breast and prostate cancer survivors (mean age 71 years) in a cross-sectional design [21]. Approximately 45% of those sampled reported meeting guidelines for vigorous exercise (at least 3 times per week for 20 min). Older cancer survivors who met criteria for vigorous exercise reported significantly higher scores on physical functioning than those not meeting guidelines. This study led to two additional home-based interventions designed to improve physical functioning among older cancer survivors.

Project LEAD randomized elders (≥65 years) within 18 months of cancer diagnosis (locoregional breast or prostate cancer) to a 6-month home-based lifestyle intervention including telephone counseling and tailored print materials designed to increase physical activity and improve overall diet [22]. Outcomes including self-reported physical function, physical activity, and diet quality were assessed at baseline, 6 and 12 months. The study recruited less than 50% of targeted enrollment due to a response rate of 34% and a large proportion of ineligible subjects, many of whom were already exercising. Among enrolled subjects, however, attrition was low. At 6 months there was a significant improvement in diet quality with a trend towards improved physical function. A second home-based intervention randomized 641 overweight older (aged 65–91) long-term survivors of colorectal, breast, and prostate cancer to telephone counseling/print materials versus a delayed intervention (control) to prompt exercise, improve diet quality, and weight loss [23]. The primary outcome of this 12-month intervention was improved self-reported physical function. The majority of subjects enrolled (mean age 73 years) were white, college educated, and had a low number of

Table 1. Randomized physical activity interventions for older cancer survivors

Reference (first author)	n	Population	Mean age	Intervention	Duration	Positive outcomes[1]	Comments
Home-based interventions							
Demark-Wahnefried [22]	182	Locoregionally staged breast and prostate survivors within 18 months of diagnosis	71	Home-based telephone counseling and print materials targeting physical activity and diet	6 months	Improved diet quality ↑ Self-efficacy for exercise	Trend towards improved self-report physical function Unable to achieve accrual target Recruitment response rate 34% Low attrition among participants
Morey [23]	641	Overweight long-term (>5 years) survivors of colorectal, breast, prostate cancer	73	Home-based telephone counseling and print materials	12 months	↑ Self-report physical function ↑ Physical activity ↑ Quality of life ↑ Weight loss	Positive response rate to mailed study invitation 11%
Payne [24]	20	Breast cancer survivors on anti-estrogen therapy	65	Home-based walking	12 weeks	Improved sleep quality	Adherence unknown due to self-report outcome
Supervised interventions							
LaStayo [25]	40	Breast, prostate, colorectal, lymphoma survivors at least 6 months post-treatment	74	Supervised progressive resistance using eccentric stepper	12 weeks	↑ Lower extremity strength ↑ 6-min walk distance ↓ Time to safely descend stairs	Recruitment response rate of 33% Excluded subjects participating in exercise
Segal[2] [26]	121	Prostate cancer patients initiating radiation therapy	66	Supervised aerobic (A) versus resistance (R)	24 weeks	↓ Fatigue (A and R) ↑ Quality of life (R) ↑ Fitness (A and R) ↑ Strength (R)	Resistance training resulted in longer term improvements compared to aerobic Recruitment rate 37% One serious adverse event (A)
Galvao[2] [30]	57	Prostate cancer patients receiving androgen suppression therapy	70	Supervised combined resistance and aerobic	12 weeks	↑ Lean mass ↑ Walk time ↑ Strength ↑ Quality of life ↓ Fatigue	Recruitment rate 59% No serious adverse events

Table 1. continued

Reference (first author)	n	Population	Mean age	Intervention	Duration	Positive outcomes[1]	Comments
Bourke[2] [29]	50	Advanced prostate cancer patients receiving androgen suppression therapy	72	Supervised and self-directed exercise (combine aerobic and resistance) and dietary advice	12 weeks	↑ Exercise behavior ↑ Aerobic tolerance ↑ Strength ↑ Diet quality	Recruitment rate 64% Supervised session attendance was high (95%) Attrition was high (44%)
Monga[2] [28]	21	Localized prostate cancer patients receiving radiation	68[3]	Supervised aerobic	8 weeks	↑ Cardiac fitness ↑ Strength ↑ Flexibility ↑ Self-report physical function and well-being	Recruitment rate 86% among eligible patients Nearly 50% screened were excluded due to comorbidity 30% enrolled subjects did not complete study

[1] $p < 0.05$.
[2] Trials were not elderly-specific but mean age >65 years.
[3] Represents mean age of exercise group, control group mean age 71 years.

comorbid conditions (mean 2) representing a selected sample of older cancer survivors. There was significantly less self-reported functional decline in the intervention group with a significant increase in targeted behaviors including exercise and improved dietary intake. Intervention subjects also reported improved quality of life. These few studies provide preliminary support for the potential benefits of home-based interventions for elderly cancer survivors and also highlight challenges related to recruitment and selection bias.

There are only a handful of small elderly-specific trials that have evaluated supervised outpatient or inpatient exercise interventions in cancer patients [24, 25] and none that have focused exclusively on elderly patients (≥65 years of age) actively receiving chemotherapy. Interventions during treatment are particularly challenging but could serve to maintain function and quality of life when patients are most vulnerable to short- and long-term disability (fig. 1). Most of the available data supporting the benefits of exercise interventions during or shortly after treatment in older cancer patients were collected in prostate cancer survivors. While these trials were

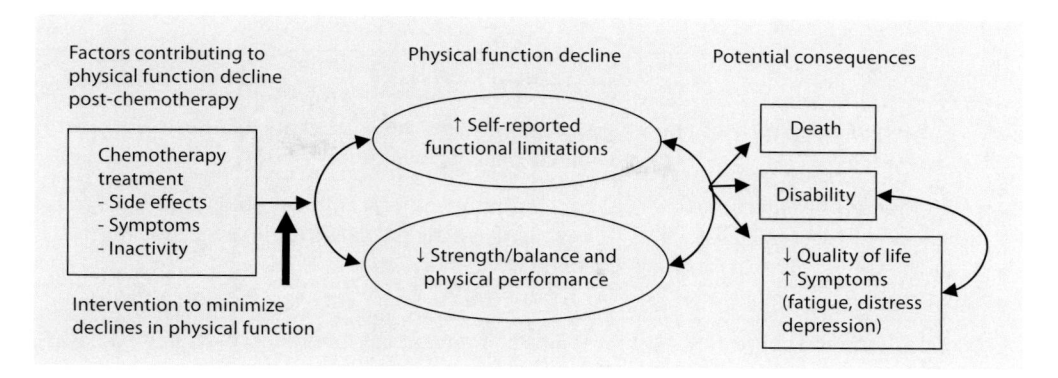

Fig. 1. Conceptual model of benefit of exercise during cancer chemotherapy treatment for older adults.

not designed as elderly-specific trials, a large proportion of patients enrolled were over 65 years of age.

Among patients receiving radiation therapy for prostate cancer, a randomized trial (mean age 66 years) of a 24-week intervention comparing supervised aerobic versus resistance training with usual care demonstrated decreased fatigue over time in both intervention arms [26]. Resistance training improved multiple secondary outcomes including quality of life, fitness, strength, and triglyceride levels with longer term improvements in symptoms seen in the resistance group compared to aerobic. Over half of the 121 subjects enrolled in this trial were over age 65. A second analysis from this trial compared outcomes by age (≤65 vs. >65 years). Older subjects appeared to derive similar benefit from exercise as younger patients enrolled in this trial. However, significant changes in body composition were only seen in the older cohort. Specifically, resistance exercise appeared to attenuate an age-related decrease in lean mass and increase in body fat which was seen in both the aerobic training and usual care arms [27]. A second study (mean age 68 for intervention group) investigating the benefit of aerobic exercise during radiation therapy showed improvements in fitness, leg strength, fatigue, and well-being compared to usual care [28]. The pilot study was limited by a small sample size and highlighted recruitment challenges when designing intervention trials for older adults. Almost half of the patients screened for this study were considered ineligible due to comorbid medical problems.

Studies have also investigated the benefit of exercise in the setting of ADT. Supervised exercise programs combining aerobic and resistance training for 12 weeks have shown positive effects on body composition (increased lean body mass), strength, walk time, as well as improved quality of life and fatigue [29, 30]. Available evidence supports the use of exercise including resistance training as a safe and effective supportive care intervention to attenuate the negative effects of ADT on body composition, strength, and function.

Table 2. Potential benefits and challenges of exercise for older cancer survivors

Potential benefits	Challenges/barriers
Positive effects on body composition (increased lean mass)	Optimal intensity, mode, duration of exercise for older cancer patients is unknown
Increased strength, flexibility, and fitness resulting in decreased risks of short- and long-term disability and increased independence	Exercise in the setting of multimorbidity and frailty has been understudied. Individualized programs are essential
Decreased fatigue and depressive symptoms	Timing of interventions for optimal benefit is unknown (i.e. during treatment versus post-treatment)
Enhanced sense of well-being, self-efficacy, and quality of life	Maintaining motivation and long-term behavior change
Improved treatment tolerance	Transportation, social support, and resources may limit long-term success of supervised exercise programs

Unique Challenges for Older Adults

Many questions remain for clinicians and patients regarding the implementation of exercise programs for older patients diagnosed with cancer (table 2). While it is clear that older patients may stand to benefit most from interventions designed to maximize functional outcomes, they also present unique challenges for the design and administration of these interventions. A primary concern is safety, particularly among frailer older adults. No safety concerns have been reported in clinical trials evaluating exercise interventions among cancer patients, including those limited trials focused specifically on an elderly cohort. Most trials, however, excluded patients with significant comorbidity such as cardiovascular disease. This limits generalizability of findings to many older adults treated for cancer who suffer from multimorbidity. In addition, most have studied longer term cancer survivors rather than newly diagnosed patients and no elderly-specific trials have investigated exercise as an adjunct to aggressive therapy (i.e. chemotherapy). Further studies among frail older cancer patients are needed to guide recommendations for this cohort in particular.

Recruitment to exercise intervention studies is a challenge as is changing physical activity behavior in clinical practice. It is unclear if willingness to participate in exercise differs significantly by age among patients with cancer, although older patients have multiple risk factors for poor participation and may be less likely to continue exercise behavior long term [31]. In addition to comorbidity, older adults are more likely to have lower levels of physical activity, worse functional status, and social limitations including transportation issues. These all represent challenges in designing and recommending practical exercise programs that can be maintained long term.

Research in non-cancer elderly populations suggests that some of these challenges can be overcome by tailoring the intervention to the individual's condition [32]. For example, the Lifestyle Interventions and Independence for Elderly Pilot (LIFE-P) randomized sedentary elderly non-cancer patients (aged 70–89) to an outpatient physical activity intervention and demonstrated both acceptable adherence to the protocol and improved physical performance at 6 and 12 months in the intervention group [32, 33]. Tailoring the intervention to the participants' baseline status could enhance efficacy [34]. Providing for flexibility in the delivery of the intervention may also be important for successful implementation in older patient populations. While supervised programs administered in controlled environments are ideal for execution of multimodal exercise activities, it may not be practical or sustainable for many older adults given competing demands on their time, transportation issues, and limitations of community resources. Simple home-based interventions may be well suited to many elders due to its practicality. Ongoing creativity will be required to develop and promote the most practical and efficient methods of exercise that can be individualized to older adult cancer patients in multiple different settings.

Conclusion

Older adults are at high risk for functional decline and impairments in quality of life after a cancer diagnosis, particularly during periods of active treatment. Exercise holds promise to attenuate declines in physical function and improve symptoms such as fatigue, distress, and depression. Available evidence demonstrates a benefit for increased physical activity among older cancer survivors and specifically among patients diagnosed and treated for prostate cancer. Few studies have focused exclusively on older adults and evidence to support exercise during chemotherapy is lacking in this population. The optimal mode, intensity, and duration of exercise are not defined for older adults with cancer and recommendations need to be individualized. Development of tailored interventions adaptable to the heterogeneous elderly population will provide much needed practical information to inform standard of care recommendations in the future.

References

1 Cruz-Jentoft AJ, Baeyens JP, Bauer JM, et al: Sarcopenia: European consensus on definition and diagnosis: Report of the European Working Group on Sarcopenia in Older People. Age Ageing 2010;39: 412–423.
2 Hawkins S, Wiswell R: Rate and mechanism of maximal oxygen consumption decline with aging: implications for exercise training. Sports Med 2003; 33:877–888.
3 Ganz PA, Guadagnoli E, Landrum MB, et al: Breast cancer in older women: quality of life and psychosocial adjustment in the 15 months after diagnosis. J Clin Oncol 2003;21:4027–4033.
4 Keating NL, Norredam M, Landrum MB, et al: Physical and mental health status of older long-term cancer survivors. J Am Geriatr Soc 2005;53: 2145–2152.

5 Sweeney C, Schmitz KH, Lazovich D, et al: Functional limitations in elderly female cancer survivors. J Natl Cancer Inst 2006;98:521–529.
6 Alibhai SM, Breunis H, Timilshina N, et al: Impact of androgen-deprivation therapy on physical function and quality of life in men with nonmetastatic prostate cancer. J Clin Oncol 2010;28:5038–5045.
7 Muss HB, Berry DA, Cirrincione C, et al: Toxicity of older and younger patients treated with adjuvant chemotherapy for node-positive breast cancer: the Cancer and Leukemia Group B Experience. J Clin Oncol 2007;25:3699–3704.
8 Midtgaard J, Baadsgaard MT, Moller T, et al: Self-reported physical activity behaviour; exercise motivation and information among Danish adult cancer patients undergoing chemotherapy. Eur J Oncol Nurs 2009;13:116–121.
9 Respini D, Jacobsen PB, Thors C, et al: The prevalence and correlates of fatigue in older cancer patients. Crit Rev Oncol Hematol 2003;47:273–279.
10 Nelson CJ, Cho C, Berk AR, et al: Are gold standard depression measures appropriate for use in geriatric cancer patients? A systematic evaluation of self-report depression instruments used with geriatric, cancer, and geriatric cancer samples. J Clin Oncol 2010;28:348–356.
11 Hurria A, Li D, Hansen K, et al: Distress in older patients with cancer. J Clin Oncol 2009;27:4346–4351.
12 Fiatarone MA, O'Neill EF, Ryan ND, et al: Exercise training and nutritional supplementation for physical frailty in very elderly people. N Engl J Med 1994; 330:1769–1775.
13 Chou CH, Hwang CL, Wu YT: Effect of exercise on physical function, daily living activities, and quality of life in the frail older adults: a meta-analysis. Arch Phys Med Rehabil 201;93:237–244.
14 Rosenbaum S, Sherrington C: Is exercise effective in promoting mental well-being in older age? A systematic review. Br J Sports Med 2011;45:1079–1080.
15 Bean JF, Vora A, Frontera WR: Benefits of exercise for community-dwelling older adults. Arch Phys Med Rehabil 2004;85:S31–S42.
16 Nelson ME, Rejeski WJ, Blair SN, et al: Physical activity and public health in older adults: recommendation from the American College of Sports Medicine and the American Heart Association. Med Sci Sports Exerc 2007;39:1435–1445.
17 Speck RM, Courneya KS, Masse LC, et al: An update of controlled physical activity trials in cancer survivors: a systematic review and meta-analysis. J Cancer Surviv 2010;4:87–100.
18 Craft LL, Vaniterson EH, Helenowski IB, et al: Exercise effects on depressive symptoms in cancer survivors: a systematic review and meta-analysis. Cancer Epidemiol Biomarkers Prev 2012;21:3–19.
19 Doyle C, Kushi LH, Byers T, et al: Nutrition and physical activity during and after cancer treatment: an American Cancer Society guide for informed choices. CA Cancer J Clin 2006;56:323–353.
20 Courneya KS, Vallance JK, McNeely ML, et al: Exercise issues in older cancer survivors. Crit Rev Oncol Hematol 2004;51:249–261.
21 Demark-Wahnfried W, Clipp EC, Morey MC, et al: Physical function and associations with diet and exercise: results of a cross-sectional survey among elders with breast or prostate cancer. Int J Behav Nutr Phys Act 2004;1:16.
22 Demark-Wahnfried W, Clipp EC, Morey MC, et al: Lifestyle intervention development study to improve physical function in older adults with cancer: outcomes from Project LEAD. J Clin Oncol 2005;24:3465–3473.
23 Morey MC, Snyder DC, Sloane R, et al: Effects of home-based diet and exercise on functional outcomes among older, overweight long-term cancer survivors: RENEW: a randomized controlled trial. JAMA 2009;301:1883–1891.
24 Payne JK, Held J, Thorpe J, et al: Effect of exercise on biomarkers, fatigue, sleep disturbances, and depressive symptoms in older women with breast cancer receiving hormonal therapy. Oncol Nurs Forum 2008;35:635–642.
25 LaStayo PC, Marcus RL, Dibble LE, et al: Eccentric exercise versus usual care with older cancer survivors: the impact on muscle and mobility – an exploratory pilot study. BMC Geriatr 2011;11:5.
26 Segal RJ, Reid RD, Courneya KS, et al: Randomized controlled trial of resistance or aerobic exercise in men receiving radiation therapy for prostate cancer. J Clin Oncol 2009;27:344–351.
27 Alberga AS, Segal RJ, Reid RD, et al: Age and androgen-deprivation therapy on exercise outcomes in men with prostate cancer. Support Care Cancer 2012;20:971–981.
28 Monga U, Garber SL, Thornby J, et al: Exercise prevents fatigue and improves quality of life in prostate cancer patients undergoing radiotherapy. Arch Phys Med Rehabil 2007;88:1416–1422.
29 Bourke L, Doll H, Crank H, et al: Lifestyle intervention in men with advanced prostate cancer receiving androgen suppression therapy: a feasibility study. Cancer Epidemiol Biomarkers Prev 2011;20: 647–657.

30 Galvao DA, Taaffe DR, Spry N, et al: Combined resistance and aerobic exercise program reverses muscle loss in men undergoing androgen suppression therapy for prostate cancer without bone metastases: a randomized controlled trial. J Clin Oncol 2010;28:340–347.

31 Courneya KS, Friedenreich CM, Reid RD, et al: Predictors of follow-up exercise behavior 6 months after a randomized trial of exercise training during breast cancer chemotherapy. Breast Cancer Res Treat 2009;114:179–187.

32 Pahor M, Blair SN, Espeland M, et al: Effects of a physical activity intervention on measures of physical performance: results of the Lifestyle Interventions and Independence for Elders Pilot (LIFE-P) study. J Gerontol A Biol Sci Med Sci 2006;61:1157–1165.

33 Rejeski WJ, Miller ME, King AC, et al: Predictors of adherence to physical activity in the Lifestyle Interventions and Independence for Elders Pilot (LIFE-P) study. Clin Interv Aging 2007;2:485–494.

34 Marsh AP, Chmelo EA, Katula JA, et al: Should physical activity programs be tailored when older adults have compromised function? J Aging Phys Act 2009;17:294–306.

Heidi D. Klepin, MD, MS
Wake Forest School of Medicine
Medical Center Blvd.
Winston-Salem, NC 27157 (USA)
E-Mail hklepin@wakehealth.edu

Aging and Cancer – Addressing a Nation's Challenge

Jeanne-Marie Bréchot · Martine Le Quellec-Nathan · Agnès Buzyn

Institut National du Cancer, Boulogne-Billancourt, France

Abstract

The incidence of cancer will increase dramatically among elderly people in the 21st century. The first French National Cancer Plan (2003–2006) with the French Ministry of Health supported the creation of 15 pilot coordination units in oncogeriatrics (UPCOG) in 13 out of the 27 French regions. The second French National Cancer Plan (2009–2013) continues to support oncogeriatrics. Based on evaluation of the pilot experiment in 2010, requirement specifications for an oncogeriatric coordination unit were defined and rolled out nationwide. The following missions were set out: to adjust cancer treatment in elderly people and enable all elderly cancer patients to benefit from this oncogeriatric approach; to stimulate specific research in oncogeriatrics; to promote training of health professionals, and to promote information. The clinical use of a geriatric prescreening tool as a routine procedure needs to become more widespread. Lastly, recommendations for treatment strategies tailored to elderly persons with high-incidence cancer must be developed. Fifteen oncogeriatrics coordination units were founded since 2011, covering 11 regions. Roll-out continues in 2012.

Copyright © 2013 S. Karger AG, Basel

In France, the estimated cancer incidence in the elderly (≥75 years) in 2011 was 65,000 (32% of all new cancer cases) in males and 52,000 (33%) in females [1]. Elderly cancer patients accounted for 29% of patients admitted to hospitals in 2010. For the whole population, cancer deaths between 2003 and 2007 were the leading cause of death in males (33%) with a median age of 72 years and the second cause of death in females (23%) with a median age of 76 years [2].

With the increase of life expectancy, half of the cancers will occur in elderly people in 2050.

Health Policy in Oncogeriatrics in France

Worldwide, the management of cancer in the elderly is gaining in portent. The benefits of a comprehensive geriatric assessment (CGA) are clearly recognized, making it possible to adapt cancer treatment and patient care to functional, emotional, socioeconomic and cognitive changes, as well as comorbidity and polymedication [3, 4]. Taking into account the growing importance of a better collaboration between oncologists and geriatricians on patient care, the first French National Cancer Plan, carried out from 2003 to 2006, dedicated one measure to oncogeriatrics. Fifteen pilot coordination units in oncogeriatrics (UPCOG) were created in 13 of the 27 regions in France and received funding.

Lessons from the Pilot Phase

An evaluation of the UPCOG's activity was conducted by the French National Cancer Institute (INCa) in 2010, after the organizations had been running for 4 or 5 years. Great heterogeneity was observed between the different pilot units. The main successful approaches were the following:

(1) Increased use of geriatric screening, either a prescreening test or a CGA. The benefit of a geriatric consultation with CGA for patients for whom treatment decisions appear subjectively complex was evaluated in one of the pilot units: for 34 patients (21%) a decrease in dose intensity or a delay was proposed and for 45 patients (27%) an increase was proposed; however, close follow-up was necessary and the vast majority of these patients required inpatient treatment. The final outcome is not yet available [5]. A very similar prospective study was conducted in another pilot unit, systematically using a CGA in 375 consecutive elderly patients with cancer and comparing the initial treatment proposal with the final treatment decision: treatment was modified in 20.8% of the patients, with a decrease of treatment intensity in the vast majority [6]. A survey evaluating the care pathway in elderly cancer patients was performed among 2,337 GPs and 481 specialist physicians and showed poor referral, worsening with patients' age, large agreement on the usefulness of a geriatric assessment, and the development of social aids at home identified as the major need [7].

(2) Clinical research dedicated to older cancer patients. As highlighted in recent publications, there is a lack of data to make evidence-based decisions with regard to chemotherapy [8], and to decide which older patients can benefit from adjuvant therapy [9]. A large multicenter open-label phase 3 randomized trial was conducted to compare a platinum-doublet chemotherapy to gemcitabine or vinorelbine monotherapy in patients aged 70–89 years with locally advanced or metastatic non-small-cell-lung cancer and demonstrated a survival benefit despite increased toxic effects with the carboplatin-paclitaxel doublet [10]. However, no CGA was performed before the

treatment, despite the well-known benefit of such an approach [11, 12]. Human and social science research was conducted in two pilot units. A qualitative social survey concluded that even in such a structure, the geriatrician's tools, expertise and know-how were often perceived ambiguously: they could be reduced to making simple assessments at the time of initial diagnosis, and their opinions and proposals often went ignored [13].

(3) The development of university training programs.

(4) Meetings, websites and papers promoting widespread information to elderly patients and their families, as well as the senior population about the improvement of cancer prognosis, even in the elderly, and the potential benefit of an appropriated treatment.

However, this pilot experience shows several limits: (a) In most UPCOGs, experience was limited to one or two healthcare institutions, or even one or two departments in these institutions. Indeed, access to a geriatrician was provided in some oncology departments, but many cancer patients continue to be addressed to academic or general hospitals and did not benefit from this organization. (b) University training in oncogeriatrics organized with the contribution of several pilot units was followed by the vast majority of geriatricians, but very few oncologists. (c) No database was set up to track the characteristics of the cancers and the patients followed in these pilot units. (d) This organization did not boost the rate of large clinical trials dedicated to this population.

Requirement Specifications of an Oncogeriatric Coordination Unit for the Next 3 Years

The second French National Cancer Plan (2009–2013), developed under the supervision of the French Ministry of Labor, Employment and Health, in conjunction with the Ministry of Higher Education and Research, continues this approach through Measure 23: 'Develop specific care management for patients with rare forms of cancer or genetic predispositions as well as for children, adolescents and the elderly'. The 23.4 action is specifically dedicated to oncogeriatrics: 'Improve care management for elderly cancer patients' and composed of three sub-actions: (1) assess the oncogeriatrics pilot coordination units and develop recommendations on setting them up nationwide; (2) finalize the clinical study on the geriatric assessment tool (Oncodage study) and expand its use beginning in 2011, and (3) develop recommendations for treatment strategies tailored to the elderly for cancers with the highest incidence, starting in 2010.

The major goal, considered as a nation's challenge, is to offer each older cancer patient appropriate care, suited to his cancer characteristics as well as his health status (age, comorbidities, long-term treatment, cognitive status...). This approach is incorporated into a global quality of care approach for all cancer patients. As a result, in France, several quality measures are now required for the authorization given to healthcare institutions to treat cancer patients. They include an announcement procedure, a multidisciplinary, individualized care plan, access to supportive care, access to innovative treatments and clinical trials, and detection of social frailty and instability.

Analysis of the pilot phase was used to define the requirements of oncogeriatrics coordination units (UCOGs) and plan their nationwide roll-out. A call for projects was launched by INCA and the Ministry of Health at the beginning of 2011, with the aim of creating one UCOG in each of the 22 metropolitan regions and the 5 overseas departments and territories. Fifteen UCOGs covering 11 regions were funded since 2011, with a global budget of EUR 3,150 million (EUR 150,000–200,000/UCOG/year); out of these, 10 participated in the pilot phase. Roll-out will continue in 2012.

These UCOGs, coordinated by an oncologist and a geriatrician (most of them MD-PhD in university hospitals authorized to treat patients with cancer), have six missions:

(1) Adjust cancer treatments for the elderly. The first step is to systematically perform a geriatric prescreening test by the oncology team for ≥75-year-old cancer patients: this will make it possible to select those who should benefit from a CGA before the treatment decision and offer appropriate geriatric support if required. The next step is a multidisciplinary discussion with the presence of a geriatrician, when needed, to discuss the treatment modalities and to choose the most appropriate cancer treatment with the optimal supportive care. In a survey conducted in five EU countries, multidisciplinary discussions about treatment patterns for elderly cancer patients were not part of standard procedure everywhere [14].

(2) Allow each elderly cancer patient to benefit from this oncogeriatric approach. It is a major challenge to prevent undertreatment in elderly patients, mostly because of age, or overtreatment, not taking into account the frailty or vulnerability, comorbidities, and polymedication. Organizing such an approach for all elderly cancer patients in a region induces close collaboration with the regional health agencies: for each region or territory coordinated by an UCOG, a list of healthcare institutions authorized to treat cancer patients and the full range of geriatric healthcare services, including mobile geriatric units, will be available for all healthcare providers in order to favor active collaboration around the patient between oncologists and geriatricians. Regional cancer networks will also participate by circulating information about cancer therapy in accordance with geriatric evaluation, the principle and the modalities of a prescreening geriatric test, access to CGA and/or geriatricians, and disseminating national guidelines dedicated to elderly patients.

(3) Stimulate specific research projects in oncogeriatrics. The development of new treatment strategies and the risks and benefits of using new drugs should be addressed in clinical trials dedicated to this population. This is critically important towards improving knowledge about appropriate cancer treatments. The National Cancer Plan targets a 5% participation rate among elderly cancer patients in clinical

trials within 5 years. UCOGs should also foster basic research, in particular studies on the biological mechanisms common to aging and cancer genesis, and humanity and social science research.

(4) Promote professional academic as well as continuous training for oncologists, geriatricians, as well as GPs, pharmacists, nurses, and mobile geriatric unit professionals.

(5) Promote information dedicated to patients, caregivers and the public. Communication should point out the benefit of a personalized treatment adjusted to the cancer and the patient, decided outside emergency situations, following appropriate evaluation of the risks and benefits; the dramatic effectiveness of some of the innovative treatments when given to the right patients (targeted therapies) should be described. The importance of participating in clinical trials should be explained to patients and their families.

(6) Implement databases enabling the prospective collection of data about the active cases in the UCOGs and describe patients and cancer characteristics. The French Society of Thoracic and Cardiovascular Surgery database, Epithor, created in 2002, with more than 135,000 procedures from 93 institutions registered, made it possible to compare the surgical treatment of lung cancer in octogenarians versus younger patients and to point out that surgical treatment should not be denied on chronological age alone [15].

Geriatric Assessment

In order to avoid the systematic need for a full CGA, the development of prescreening tools validated for cancer patients appears essential. Therefore, CGA should be offered to selected patients, but according to objective criteria. A preliminary study conducted in the Bordeaux pilot unit evaluated the G-8 screening tool: with a cut-off value of 14, it showed good screening properties for identifying elderly cancer patients who could benefit from CGA [16].

Following this preliminary study, a multicenter prospective study was conducted in France (and funded by INCa) between 2008 and 2010 to validate the G-8 screening geriatric tool in cancer patients (ASCO 2011). Most of the pilot units participated; 1,668 patients were included, 1,590 were eligible, and 1,425 deemed suitable for evaluation. The 8 items tool (G-8) was confirmed to be quick and easy to perform. Abnormal G-8 was observed in 68.4% of the 1,425 patients, and abnormal CGA was observed in 80.1%. Compared to CGA, its sensitivity was 76.6%, 95% CI 74–79% and its specificity 64.4%, 95% CI 58.6–70.0%. Therefore, the G-8 can be used as a screening tool before treatment for cancer patients older than 70, making it possible to predict at least one abnormal CGA test among the Cumulative Illness Rating Scale for Geriatrics (CIRS-G), Activities of Daily Living (ADL) and Instrumental Activities of Daily Living (IADL) questionnaires, the Mini-Mental

Status Examination (MMSE), the Mini-Nutritional Assessment (MNA), the Geriatric Depression Scale (GDS-15) and the 'Timed Get Up and Go' evaluation [17].

The use of this screening tool is expanding in France. However, as this study has not been published yet, some UCOGs currently recommend other geriatric tools, such as the Vulnerable Elders Survey (VES-13).

Conclusion

The organization of oncogeriatrics in France is a real challenge for several reasons: (1) Oncogeriatrics is neither a new specialty nor a new healthcare setting. It is based on active collaboration between oncologists and geriatricians, fostering more global improvement of the quality of care for cancer patients. Announcement procedures, multidisciplinary treatment planning meetings, and the definition of criteria making it possible to set up an authorization framework for the delivery of cancer care services are some of the key milestones of this quality process. (2) Clinical research dedicated to elderly cancer patients must be developed, making it possible to evaluate the benefit-risk ratio of standard or innovative treatments, taking into account the specificities of this population. Research in some other aspects, particularly social or ethical, such as advance guidelines (making it possible for competent patients to record the nature and type of medical procedures they wish to receive, should they become incompetent) must be developed [18].

References

1 Projection de l'incidence et de la mortalité par cancer en France en 2011. Rapport technique. Saint-Maurice: Institut de veille sanitaire, 2011. 78p. Disponible à partir de l'URL: http://www.invs.sante.fr.
2 Dynamique d'évolution des taux de mortalité des principaux cancers en France: Rapports et synthèses, novembre 2010, Institut national du cancer: www.e-cancer.fr.
3 Balducci L, Extermann M: Management of cancer in the older person: a practical approach. Oncologist 2000;5:224–237.
4 Extermann M, Hurria A: Comprehensive geriatric assessment for older patients with cancer. J Clin Oncol 2007;14:1824–1831.
5 Chaïbi P, Magné N, Breton S, et al: Influence of geriatric consultation with comprehensive geriatric assessment on final therapeutic decision in elderly cancer patients. Crit Rev Oncol Hematol 2011;79:302–307.
6 Caillet P, Canoui-Poitrine F, Vouriot J, et al: Comprehensive geriatric assessment in the decision-making process in elderly patients with cancer: ELCAPA study. J Clin Oncol 2011;29:3636–3642.
7 Kurtz J-E, Heitz D, Enderlin P, et al: Geriatric oncology, general practitioners and specialists: current opinions and unmet needs. Crit Rev Oncol Hematol 2010;75:47–57.
8 Lichtman SM, Wieldiers H, Chatelut E, et al: International Society of Geriatric Oncology Chemotherapy Taskforce: evaluation of chemotherapy in older patients – an analysis of the medical literature. J Clin Oncol 2007;25:1832–1843.
9 Muss HB, Biganzoli L, Sargent DJ, Aapro M: Adjuvant therapy in the elderly: making the right decision. J Clin Oncol 2007;25:1870–1875.

10 Quoix E, Zalcman G, Oster JP, et al, Intergroupe Francophone de Cancérologie Thoracique: Carboplatin and weekly paclitaxel doublet chemotherapy compared with monotherapy in elderly patients with advanced non-small-cell lung cancer: IFCT-0501 randomized phase 3 trial. Lancet 2011;378: 1079–1088.

11 Droz J-P, Aapro M, Balducci L: Overcoming challenges associated with chemotherapy treatment in the senior adult population. Crit Rev Oncol Hematol 2008;68(suppl):S1–S8.

12 Hurria A, Togawa K, Mohile SG, et al: Predicting chemotherapy toxicity in older adults with cancer: a prospective multicenter study. J Clin Oncol 2011; 29:3457–3465.

13 Sifer-Rivière L, Girre V, Gisselbrecht M, Saint-Jean O: Physicians' perceptions of cancer care for elderly patients: a qualitative sociological study based on a pilot geriatric oncology program. Crit Rev Oncol Hematol 2010;75:58–69.

14 Anhoury P, Pickhaert A-P, Ramsey B, et al: The European oncologist approach to geriatric patients (abstract). Crit Rev Oncol Hematol 2009; 72(suppl 1):S19.

15 Rivera C, Dahan M, Bernard A, et al: Surgical treatment of lung cancer in the octogenarians: results of a nationwide audit. Eur J Cardiothorac Surg 2011;39:981–986.

16 Bellera CA, Rainfray M, Mathoulin-Pélissier S, et al: Screening older cancer patients: first evaluation of the G-8 geriatric screening tool. Ann Oncol 2012; 23:2166–2172.

17 Soubeyran P, Bellera C, Goyard J, et al: Validation of the G-8 screening tool in geriatric oncology: the Oncodage project. J Clin Oncol 2011;29(suppl): abstr 9001.

18 Pautex S, Notaridis G, Déramé L, Zulian GB: Preferences of elderly cancer patients in their advance directives. Crit Rev Oncol Hematol 2010;74:61–65.

Dr. Jeanne-Marie Bréchot
Institut National du Cancer
52, avenue Morizet
FR–92513 Boulogne-Billancourt
E-Mail jmbrechot@institutcancer.fr

Author Index

Albrand, G. 132
Audisio, R.A. 124

Balducci, L. 61
Bréchot, J.-M. 158
Buzyn, A. 158

Campisi, J. 17
Curiel, T.J. 1

Demaria, M. 17

Extermann, M. VII, 49

Fulop, T. 38

Gravekamp, C. 28

Holmes, H.M. 132
Huisman, M.G. 124

Klepin, H.D. 146

Kotb, R. 38

Larbi, A. 38
Le Quellec-Nathan, M. 158
Lichtman, S.M. 104
Livi, C.B. 1

Magnuson, A. 85
Mihalko, S. 146
Mohile, S.G. 85, 146

Overcash, J. 139

Pawelec, G. 38

Sharp, Z.D. 1

van Leeuwen, B.L. 124
Velarde, M.C. 17
Vey, N. 73

Subject Index

Activities of daily living, frailty assessment 63, 64, 68
Acute myeloid leukemia
   elderly patients
      clinical manifestations 75–77
      host-disease interactions 77–79
      management 79–82
      risk stratification 80, 81
   epidemiology 73
   genetics 74, 75
   treatment overview 73, 74
Adaptive immunity
   cancer patients 30, 31
   cancer vaccination optimization 33–36
   elderly 29, 40–42, 44
   metabolic syndrome and cancer risk 53
Adiponectin, metabolic syndrome and cancer risk 53
Advanced glycation end-products, metabolic syndrome and cancer risk 51, 52
Aging
   cancer relationship 3, 17, 18, 38
   cancer vaccination in elderly, *see* Cancer vaccination
   cellular senescence, *see* Senescence, cellular
   demographics 3
   frailty, *see* Frailty
   immune response, *see* Adaptive immunity, Immunosenescence, Innate immunity
Anthracyclines, pharmacology in older patients 111

Bendamustine, pharmacology in older patients 107

Caloric restriction, *see* Diet restriction

Cancer vaccination
   adaptive immunity
      cancer patients 30, 31
      elderly 29
   innate immunity
      cancer patients 31, 32
      elderly 29, 30
   preclinical studies in old animals 32, 33
Capecitabine, pharmacology in older patients 108, 109
Carboplatin, pharmacology in older patients 110, 111
Cardiovascular Health Study, frailty phenotype 64–68
Cellular senescence, *see* Senescence, cellular
Chemotherapy pharmacology, *see* specific drugs, Pharmacology
Cisplatin, pharmacology in older patients 110
Comprehensive Geriatric Assessment
   components
      cognition 90, 91
      comorbidity 88, 89
      functional status 86–88
      geriatric syndromes 93
      nutrition 91
      objective physical performance 88
      polypharmacy 89, 90
      psychological distress 92, 93
      social support and finances 91, 92
   frailty assessment 63, 64, 70
   French coordination units in oncogeriatrics 162, 164
   nurse's role 141, 142
   outcome improvement in older cancer patients 97, 98
   overview 85, 86

risk stratification 93–95
Coordination units in oncogeriatrics, see France, oncogeriatrics
Cyclophosphamide, pharmacology in older patients 107
Cytarabine, pharmacology in older patients 114

Diet restriction, mechanistic target of rapamycin relationship 4, 6, 7
Docetaxel, pharmacology in older patients 113

Economic impact, cancer 1, 2
eRapa, see Rapamycin
Etoposide, pharmacology in older patients 115, 116
Exercise
　benefits in elderly without cancer 148, 149
　cancer survivors
　　non-elderly 149, 150
　　older cancer patients 150–154
　cancer treatment effects on physical function and well-being 147, 148
　challenges in elderly 154, 155
　functional decline after cancer diagnosis 147

5-Fluorouracil
　patient age effects on toxicity 108
　pharmacology in older patients 107, 108
Fludarabine, pharmacology in older patients 114
Frailty
　cancer association 70
　clinical definition
　　indices 68, 69
　　phenotype 64–68
　　physiologic age assessment 62–64
　　vulnerability 69
　overview 61, 62
France, oncogeriatrics
　coordination units in oncogeriatrics establishment 159
　geriatric assessment 162, 163
　pilot phase 159, 160
　requirement specification 160–162
　demographics 158
　prospects 163

G8, geriatric oncology utilization 96, 97
Gemcitabine, pharmacology in older patients 114
Geriatrician
　education gaps 137
　incorporation into oncology 135, 136
　overlap with oncology 133
　partnerships in geriatrics and oncology 134–136
　shortages 134
Groningen Frailty Indicator, geriatric oncology utilization 96

Immune response, see Adaptive immunity, Innate immunity
Immune surveillance
　immunosenescence and immunoediting 20
　tumorigenesis prevention 39
　tumors and immunoediting 8, 9
Immunosenescence
　cancer relationship 42–44
　overview 20, 40–42
　restoration of immune function in aging 45
Immunotherapy, see Cancer vaccination
Inflammation, metabolic syndrome and cancer risk 53
Innate immunity
　cancer patients 31, 32
　elderly 29, 30, 40, 43
Instrumental activities of daily living, frailty assessment 63, 64, 68
Insulin-like growth factor-1, metabolic syndrome and cancer risk 50, 51
Insulin resistance, metabolic syndrome and cancer risk 51
Intervention Testing Program 3–5
Irinotecan, pharmacology in older patients 115

Leptin, metabolic syndrome levels and cancer risk 53

Mage-b, DNA vaccine 33
Mammalian target of rapamycin, see Mechanistic target of rapamycin
Mechanistic target of rapamycin
　comparative biology 5
　diet restriction response 4, 6, 7
　downstream effectors 5, 6

functional overview 3, 4
inhibition
 cancer prevention 10–13
 clinical trials 10, 11
 immune modulation 9
 metformin 11
lifespan modulation 6
Melphalan, pharmacology in older patients 106, 107
Metabolic syndrome, cancer risk
 animal studies 54, 55
 clinical trials 55, 56
 epidemiology 49, 50
 mechanisms 50–54
Metformin
 cancer prevention 55
 mechanistic target of rapamycin inhibition 11
Myeloid-derived suppressor cell 31, 35

Nursing, geriatric oncology
 functions
  advocacy for patient and family 142, 143
  Comprehensive Geriatric Assessment 141, 142
  education of patient and family 142
  research 143, 144
 multidisciplinary team composition and function 140, 141
 overview 139

Oncological surgery, see Surgery, oncogeriatric
Oncologist
 education gaps 137
 incorporation into geriatrics 137
 overlap with geriatrics 133
 partnerships in geriatrics and oncology 134–136
 shortages 133
Oxiplatin, pharmacology in older patients 109, 110

Paclitaxel, pharmacology in older patients 112, 113
Pemetrexed, pharmacology in older patients 114
Peroxisome proliferator-activated receptor, metabolic syndrome activity and cancer risk 54

Pharmacology, see also specific drugs
 alkylating agents 106
 antimicrotubule agents 111, 112
 camptothecans 115, 116
 platinum compounds 109–111
 prospects for study in elderly 116, 117
 purine analogs 114
 rationale for study in older patients 105, 106
 taxanes 112, 113
Physical activity, see Exercise
Postoperative cognitive dysfunction 126, 127
Protein kinase C-ζ, metabolic syndrome activation and cancer risk 51–53
PTEN, mutation and cancer 21

Rapamycin, see also Mechanistic target of rapamycin
 antifungal activity 10
 cancer trials 12
 eRapa studies 6, 9, 10, 12
 immunosuppression 9, 10
 mechanisms of lifespan and cancer mediation 7, 8

Senescence, cellular, see also Immunosenescence
 aging 18
 anti-senescence-associated secretory phenotype therapy for cancer 22–24
 senescence-associated secretory phenotype 19, 20, 24, 245
 senescence-elimination therapy for cancer 24
 senescence-induction therapy for cancer 21, 22
 stimuli 18
 tumor promotion and progression
  cell proliferation 20
  immunosenescence and immunoediting 20
 tumor suppression
  cell autonomous tumor suppression 19
  non-cell autonomous tumor suppression 19
 overview 18
Surgery, oncogeriatric
 alternative treatments 128, 129
 complications in postoperative period 127, 128

education and training 129
  outcomes 126, 127
  preoperative decision-making 124–126

Topotecan, pharmacology in older
  patients 115
Tumor vaccine, *see* Cancer vaccination

Vincristine, pharmacology in older
  patients 111, 112
Vulnerability, frailty 69
Vulnerable Elders Survey-13, geriatric
  oncology utilization 95